D0604100

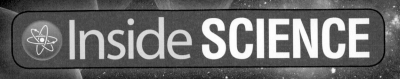

Vaccine Research

Other titles in the *Inside Science* series:

Inside SCIENCE

Vaccine Research

Toney Allman

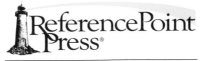

ReferencePoint
Press®

San Diego, CA

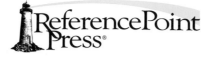

© 2011 ReferencePoint Press, Inc.

For more information, contact:
ReferencePoint Press, Inc.
PO Box 27779
San Diego, CA 92198
www. ReferencePointPress.com

LIBRARY OF CONGRESS CATALOGING-IN-PUBLICATION DATA

Allman, Toney.
Vaccine research: by toney allman.
    p. cm. — (Inside science)
Includes bibliographical references and index.
ISBN-13: 978-1-60152-131-6 (hardback)
ISBN-10: 1-60152-131-6 (hardback)
1. Vaccines—Popular works. I. Title.
QR189.A375 2011
615'.372—dc22

                                                                    2010020635

Contents

Foreword

In 2008, when the Yale Project on Climate Change and the George Mason University Center for Climate Change Communication asked Americans, "Do you think that global warming is happening?" 71 percent of those polled—a significant majority—answered "yes." When the poll was repeated in 2010, only 57 percent of respondents said they believed that global warming was happening. Other recent polls have reported a similar shift in public opinion about climate change.

Although respected scientists and scientific organizations worldwide warn that a buildup of greenhouse gases, mainly caused by human activities, is bringing about potentially dangerous and long-term changes in Earth's climate, it appears that doubt is growing among the general public. What happened to bring about this change in attitude over such a short period of time? Climate change skeptics claim that scientists have greatly overstated the degree and the dangers of global warming. Others argue that powerful special interests are minimizing the problem for political gain. Unlike experiments conducted under strictly controlled conditions in a lab or petri dish, scientific theories, facts, and findings on such a critical topic as climate change are often subject to personal, political, and media bias—whether for good or for ill.

At its core, however, scientific research is not about politics or 30-second sound bites. Scientific research is about questions and measurable observations. Science is the process of discovery and the means for developing a better understanding of ourselves and the world around us. Science strives for facts and conclusions unencumbered by bias, distortion, and political sensibilities. Although sometimes the methods and motivations are flawed, science attempts to develop a body of knowledge that can guide decision makers, enhance daily life, and lay a foundation to aid future generations.

The relevance and the implications of scientific research are profound, as members of the National Academy of Sciences point out in the 2009 edition of *On Being a Scientist: A Guide to Responsible Conduct in Research:*

Some scientific results directly affect the health and well-being of individuals, as in the case of clinical trials or toxicological studies. Science also is used by policy makers and voters to make informed decisions on such pressing issues as climate change, stem cell research, and the mitigation of natural hazards. . . . And even when scientific results have no immediate applications—as when research reveals new information about the universe or the fundamental constituents of matter—new knowledge speaks to our sense of wonder and paves the way for future advances.

The *Inside Science* series provides students with a sense of the painstaking work that goes into scientific research—whether its focus is microscopic cells cultured in a lab or planets far beyond the solar system. Each book in the series examines how scientists work and where that work leads them. Sometimes, the results are positive. Such was the case for Edwin McClure, a once-active high school senior diagnosed with multiple sclerosis, a degenerative disease that leads to difficulties with coordination, speech, and mobility. Thanks to stem cell therapy, in 2009 a healthier McClure strode across a stage to accept his diploma from Virginia Commonwealth University. In some cases, cutting-edge experimental treatments fail with tragic results. This is what occurred in 1999 when 18-year-old Jesse Gelsinger, born with a rare liver disease, died four days after undergoing a newly developed gene therapy technique. Such failures may temporarily halt research, as happened in the Gelsinger case, to allow for investigation and revision. In this and other instances, however, research resumes, often with renewed determination to find answers and solve problems.

Through clear and vivid narrative, carefully selected anecdotes, and direct quotations each book in the *Inside Science* series reinforces the role of scientific research in advancing knowledge and creating a better world. By developing an understanding of science, the responsibilities of the scientist, and how scientific research affects society, today's students will be better prepared for the critical challenges that await them. As members of the National Academy of Sciences state: "The values on which science is based—including honesty, fairness, collegiality, and openness—serve as guides to action in everyday life as well as in research. These values have helped produce a scientific enterprise of unparalleled usefulness, productivity, and creativity. So long as these values are honored, science—and the society it serves—will prosper."

Important Events in Vaccine Research

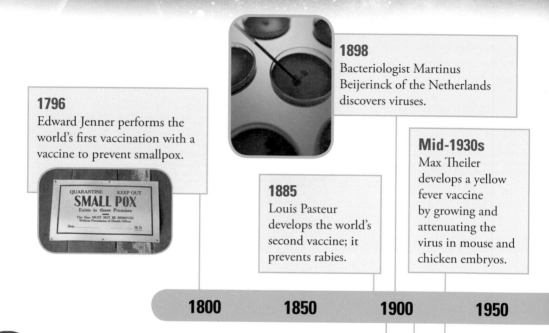

1796
Edward Jenner performs the world's first vaccination with a vaccine to prevent smallpox.

1898
Bacteriologist Martinus Beijerinck of the Netherlands discovers viruses.

Mid-1930s
Max Theiler develops a yellow fever vaccine by growing and attenuating the virus in mouse and chicken embryos.

1885
Louis Pasteur develops the world's second vaccine; it prevents rabies.

| 1800 | 1850 | 1900 | 1950 |

1890
German scientist Emil von Behring discovers that animals injected with toxins from diphtheria bacteria develop antitoxins in their blood that protect them against diphtheria infection.

1908
Paul Ehrlich is awarded the Nobel Prize in Physiology or Medicine for his research on the immune system and his description of the "magic bullets"—antibodies—that seek out and destroy invaders.

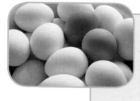

1931
At Vanderbilt University in Tennessee, pathologist Ernest Goodfellow discovers a method of growing large amounts of viruses in the laboratory by using fertilized chicken eggs.

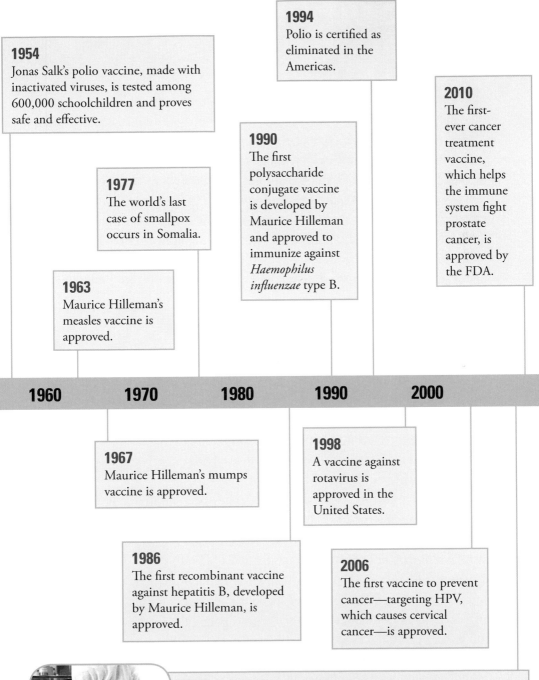

1954
Jonas Salk's polio vaccine, made with inactivated viruses, is tested among 600,000 schoolchildren and proves safe and effective.

1994
Polio is certified as eliminated in the Americas.

2010
The first-ever cancer treatment vaccine, which helps the immune system fight prostate cancer, is approved by the FDA.

1977
The world's last case of smallpox occurs in Somalia.

1990
The first polysaccharide conjugate vaccine is developed by Maurice Hilleman and approved to immunize against *Haemophilus influenzae* type B.

1963
Maurice Hilleman's measles vaccine is approved.

1960   **1970**   **1980**   **1990**   **2000**

1967
Maurice Hilleman's mumps vaccine is approved.

1998
A vaccine against rotavirus is approved in the United States.

1986
The first recombinant vaccine against hepatitis B, developed by Maurice Hilleman, is approved.

2006
The first vaccine to prevent cancer—targeting HPV, which causes cervical cancer—is approved.

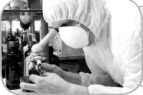

2009
Researchers with the International AIDS Vaccine Initiative discover two new antibodies for HIV (the virus that causes AIDS) in the blood of a person in Africa.

To Save Lives

On March 31, 2009, a 10-year-old boy showed up at the San Diego Naval Medical Center, sick with influenza. Medical tests could not identify the type of flu virus infecting the child. In April a 9-year-old girl living in Brawley, California, was also found to be ill with an unknown flu virus. Samples from both children were sent to the Centers for Disease Control and Prevention (CDC) to be analyzed and identified. At around the same time, doctors in Mexico City were coping with a mysterious flu epidemic that was bringing about 35 to 50 people a day to hospital emergency rooms with breathing problems, and some of these people were dying. Samples from these people, too, were sent to the CDC. Scientists at the CDC discovered to their horror that all of these infections were caused by exactly the same virus; a new kind of influenza was infecting people hundreds of miles apart and, unlike the usual seasonal flu, there was no vaccine to prevent its spread.

By June 11, 2009, this virus, now identified as swine flu or H1N1, was infecting people in at least 70 different countries and was declared a pandemic by the World Health Organization (WHO). Vaccine makers rushed to develop a vaccine that could protect against H1N1. WHO and the CDC feared that millions of infections would occur if the virus spread. In the fall of 2009, the first batches of a vaccine to prevent the H1N1 flu virus were available, but only in a limited supply. By March 2010 WHO reported at least 16,813 confirmed H1N1 deaths worldwide in 213 countries. In Africa, in countries such as Nigeria, Senegal, South Africa, and Kenya, H1N1 cases were still increasing in the spring of 2010, even as the flu season was winding down in other parts of the world. These countries had never had access to the new H1N1 vaccine because of cost and distribution problems.

> **pandemic**
>
> Epidemic of disease that is widespread and prevalent throughout an entire country, a continent, or the world.

Vaccines Needed

An ample and readily available H1N1 vaccine might have saved thousands of lives, but protecting people from infection and disease is not always easy. Vaccines have saved millions of lives around the world, and yet WHO estimates that at least 4.1 million people, the majority of them children, die each year from vaccine-preventable diseases. This includes deaths not just from new diseases, such as H1N1, but also from ones conquered long ago in wealthy countries. For example, about 500,000 children still die of measles every year, 95 percent of them in poor, underdeveloped countries, such as in parts of Africa and Asia, and mainly because the cost of vaccines and vaccine distribution is more than most of these countries can afford.

The desire to prevent suffering and premature death is the driving force behind vaccine research. The CDC explains: "Disease prevention is the key to public health. It is always better to prevent a disease than to treat it. Vaccines prevent disease in the people who receive them and protect those who come into contact with unvaccinated individuals."[1]

Masked patients with flu-like symptoms wait outside a Mexico City hospital emergency room in April 2009, as the country's influenza epidemic builds. Hospitals saw dozens of ill patients with similar symptoms every day around this time period.

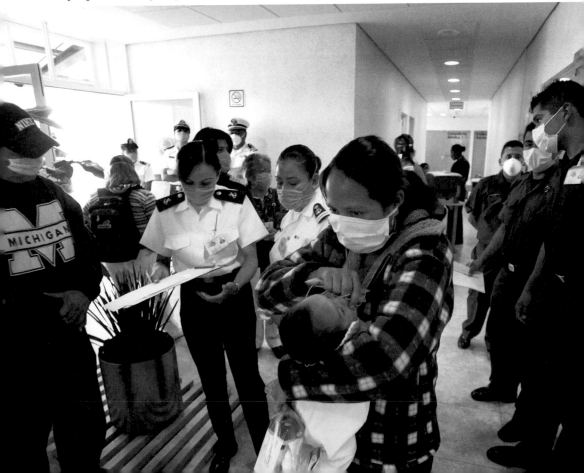

A vaccinated person usually cannot get the disease specific to that vaccine and, just as importantly, cannot spread infection to other people. In the United States and other developed countries, widespread vaccination has controlled many infectious diseases, including polio, measles, diphtheria, pertussis (whooping cough), rubella (German measles), mumps, and tetanus. These diseases were common in the past but are no longer a threat to public health, thanks to vaccine research and development. Eliminating these diseases worldwide requires universal vaccination programs, and conquering other killer diseases depends upon the development of new vaccines.

The director of the Queensland Institute of Medical Research in Australia, Michael Good, explains the motivation behind today's vaccine research:

> Learning how to harness the power of the immune system to combat infectious killers has been one of the most dramatic developments in the history of medicine. Eradication of smallpox and the near elimination of polio serve to remind us that the destiny of disease can be written by human ingenuity. These and other great feats continue to inspire us all as we strive to combat major infectious killers of the 21st Century. . . . The consequences of not doing so are too awful to contemplate.[2]

What Are Vaccines?

Jeryl Lynn Hilleman was five years old when she got the mumps. It was 1963 and, like about half of the children of her generation, Jeryl Lynn would suffer through a week or two of symptoms such as fever, body aches, weakness, painful swallowing, and swollen salivary glands that puffed up her cheeks like a chipmunk's. There were no medicines to heal the mumps and no medical treatments to prevent infection by the virus. At that time, about 1 million people in the United States caught the mumps every year. Most recovered with no problems, as did Jeryl Lynn, but for some the outcome was not so benign. Rarely—in less than 1 percent of cases—children became seriously ill as the mumps attacked their brains and spinal cords, and this complication could cause permanent paralysis or deafness. Adults faced greater risks, with about 15 percent facing brain and spinal cord involvement. In about 25 percent of adult men, the testicles were attacked by the virus, and this could cause sterility. Mumps infections doubled the risk of miscarriage in pregnant women.

Most people thought of mumps as something best gotten over with in childhood because most children would not only recover easily but also never be able to catch the mumps again. They would be protected from reinfection for the rest of their lives. As adults, therefore, they would not risk complications and permanent damage from getting the mumps.

Immunity Without Sickness

Jeryl Lynn's father, however, viewed her sickness in an entirely different way. Unlike many people, Maurice Hilleman was aware that mumps could be dangerous, even for children. Hilleman was a chemist and microbiologist who worked at Merck & Co. and specialized in developing vaccines. He worried about his daughter, but since he could not change the fact of her infection, he decided instead to use the opportunity of her illness to help others and develop a vaccine that would prevent mumps from sickening anyone else. Toward that end, Hilleman rubbed a cotton swab along the back of Jeryl Lynn's throat in order to capture the pathogen—the disease-causing agent—that causes mumps. In this case the pathogen was a virus. Hilleman's challenge was to figure out how to grow the virus and then make it safe for human bodies. He would then use it as a vaccine to prevent mumps. The vaccine would prevent the disease by teaching the body's immune system to recognize and fight off the virus. The National Institute of Allergy and Infectious Diseases explains, "Vaccines . . . trick the body into thinking an infection has occurred."[3] Once this happens, whether or not the pathogen caused actual sickness, the person is protected against reinfection because the immune system, in a sense, knows how to fight the pathogen.

> **pathogen**
>
> Any bacterium, virus, or other microorganism that causes disease.

The immune system is the body's very complex network of defenses against the myriad pathogens—viruses, bacteria, parasites, and fungi—that threaten the body's health and well-being. People are under almost constant attack from these foreign invaders, yet most of the time pathogens are fought off so successfully that people are unaware that an invasion has taken place. Only when an all-out immune system battle is required do people experience symptoms and know that they are sick. That is because a complete immune system defense takes time to launch and because the attack may be so overwhelming that the immune system cannot respond well enough to prevent disease and damage. Vaccines avoid these problems by presenting the immune system with a pathogen so weak and helpless that it is easily conquered. Then, having been "educated" about the particular pathogen in the vaccine, the immune system remembers the invader and can mount an instant defense should it ever attack again. Vaccines could do nothing, however, without marshaling the forces of the body's natural immune system defenses.

The Innate Immune System: It Just Knows

The immune system is so complicated that it is still not fully understood, but scientists have learned much about its function. The first lines of defense for the immune system are the physical barriers of the skin and the mucous membranes that line the body systems that are exposed to the outside world. Mucous membranes are found in reproductive organs, the digestive system (for example, in the mouth, stomach, and intestines), and respiratory system (for example, in the nose and lungs). In many instances these barriers alone prevent foreign substances, germs, and other pathogens from gaining access to the body. If, however, these barriers are breached, the second line of defense must take action. It is called the innate immune system. The innate immune system is composed of different kinds of specialized white blood cells that originate in the bone marrow, in the centers of bones, where all blood cells are made. Some of these innate immune system cells specialize in punching holes in bacteria; others can kill bacteria, viruses, parasites, and even some cancer cells; still others help to marshal all the forces of the immune system when an invasion is serious. One basic defending cell of the innate immune system is the macrophage.

Throughout the body, just under the surface of membranes and the skin, lie the macrophages, the all-important sentinels of the innate

In 1957, as midwestern states experienced the worst mumps outbreak in more than 20 years, the parents of one Illinois boy posted a sign warning friends of his condition. Until the development of a vaccine, mumps afflicted about 1 million Americans each year.

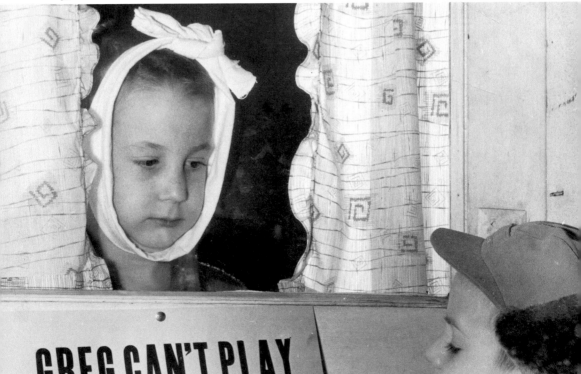

GREG CAN'T PLAY
MUMPS

immune system. Macrophages are produced in the marrow and travel through the bloodstream to their positions, where most of the time they are in a resting state. However, they have the innate, or inborn, ability to detect the foreign molecules of common invaders with what might be thought of as antennae—receptors on the surfaces of the macrophage cell. Once alerted to the invader, a macrophage moves toward it and eats it. Inside the macrophage is a pouch of dangerous chemicals that destroy the pathogen. Often, when the invasion is a small one, the macrophages handle things on their own, but sometimes help is needed. Biology professor and immune system expert

The Godfather of Modern Vaccines

Maurice Hilleman was born on August 30, 1919, on a Montana farm. Both his mother and his twin sister died at his birth. Hilleman always said he had cheated death. He was raised by relatives and lived a poor, hardworking existence, but he loved science and wanted an education. He received a scholarship to Montana State University and then attended the University of Chicago, receiving a doctorate in virology and microbiology in 1944. At that time, academics were scornful of industry, and Hilleman's advisors insisted that he become a university professor. Hilleman refused to conform to expectations and chose the pharmaceutical industry. He explained, "I wanted to do something. I wanted to make things!" And he believed that a scientist should serve society.

At Merck & Co., Hilleman served society with his vaccine research. During his long career, he developed or codeveloped about three dozen vaccines. Other scientists described him as the godfather of modern vaccines, saying he saved more lives than any other scientist of the twentieth century. At the end of his life, Hilleman was working on a vaccine for the cancer that was killing him, and he was testing the vaccine on himself. His research was cut short when he died on April 11, 2005. Few people around the world know Hilleman's name. He never named a vaccine after himself or sought praise. He said he was too busy looking for the next lifesaving vaccine.

Quoted in Paul A. Offit, *Vaccinated: One Man's Quest to Defeat the World's Deadliest Diseases.* New York: HarperCollins, 2008, p. 11.

Lauren Sompayrac explains that macrophages constantly "check for invaders." Then, he says, "When these sentinels encounter the enemy, they send out [chemical] signals that recruit more defenders to the site of the battle. The macrophages then do their best to hold off these invaders until reinforcements arrive."[4]

The Adaptive Immune System: It Learns

In an invasion such as the mumps virus, for example, blood cells from the adaptive immune system are necessary to win the battle. The adaptive immune system consists of several different kinds of white blood cells that can adapt and change themselves in response to a specific pathogen in order to defeat it. The most important of these cells are B cells and T cells. Macrophages recognize common pathogens, but they do not recognize unusual pathogens that invade the body, and they are unable to detect and eat pathogens that get inside human body cells. They can attack and kill common microbes, the tiny one-celled living organisms visible only under a microscope, such as bacteria, but they cannot defeat a large parasitic worm nor single-handedly fight an unusual bacterium, such as the one that causes whooping cough (pertussis). They also are not good at defending against viruses because viruses are able to penetrate cells where macrophages cannot find them. Once inside cells, viruses force the cells to help them reproduce—make more viruses through the process of copying and cell division. Eventually, the multiplying viruses explode out of the body cell, killing it, and go on to infect more cells. Macrophages cannot destroy the viruses inside cells, but they can detect dead and dying cells. They can attack the viruses that have not yet made it into cells. In both situations, macrophages and other cells in the innate immune system deliver chemical alarm signals to the adaptive immune system, indicating that help is needed.

antigens

Any substances or molecules that provoke an immune system response and the production of antibodies.

One way this happens is that innate immune system cells carry pieces of battle material to a lymph node. This material is often foreign proteins that are on the surfaces of invaders. These foreign substances are called antigens. An antigen is anything that can trigger an immune system response. Billions of B cells live in the lymph nodes and bloodstream. Given the right signals,

B cells are able to produce antibodies—protein molecules that act like hands that can grasp, or bind to, antigens and mark them for destruction. Scientists estimate that the B cells of the human body are capable of recognizing 100 million different kinds of antigens—enough to protect against every possible invader. However, different B cells have many different kinds of "hands," in order to be able to bind with all the many different kinds of disease antigens that might attack humans. Of the 3 billion B cells in the body, only about 30 can recognize any specific antigen. Sompayrac explains, "Said another way, although we have B cells in our arsenal that can deal with essentially any invader, we don't have a lot of any one kind of B cell. As a result, when we are attacked, more of the appropriate B cells must be made."[5] This is exactly what B cells that bind with antigens do. These experienced or educated B cells quickly begin to make more of themselves. Through a process of cell growth and division, the B cell specific to the antigen proliferates, or makes many more experienced B cells. After about a week, this one B cell will have multiplied to 20,000 cells.

> ### antibodies
>
> Immune system proteins produced on the surfaces of B cells that respond to foreign substances or antigens. A particular antibody binds to a specific antigen and tags it for destruction.

Marked for Destruction

The antibodies swarm out of the lymph node and travel through the bloodstream to the site of the infection. The job of all these antibodies, explains Sompayrac, is to mark the invaders for destruction. Scientists say that antibodies opsonize invaders, which literally means "prepare them for eating." Sompayrac suggests that it is easier to think of the antibodies as decorating viruses and bacteria. Antibodies bind to the invaders and hang on to and decorate their surfaces. Antibodies also can bind to viruses outside of cells and prevent them from entering cells. This keeps the viruses available for eating. They can neutralize the toxins, or poisons, that are produced by some bacterial invaders. They chemically signal different parts of the innate immune system to activate and start killing invaders. They can form a chemical bridge between macrophages and invaders so that macrophages will recognize and eat even uncommon viruses and bacteria. When this

> ### opsonize
>
> Decorate with antibodies in order to mark for destruction.

happens, macrophages also display the antigens of the invaders on their surfaces, signaling to the immune system's other players what is going on.

A trillion T cells of various kinds wait to be called to action in the human body. One important kind, called helper T cells, can read the chemical messages from macrophages and other immune system fighters—the specific antigens of the invasion. Helper T cells direct other cells' responses. One of the major jobs of helper T cells is to communicate with B cells. This chemical signaling helps determine how big an attack should be launched. Helper T cells can stimulate more and more B cells to make antibodies if an infection is severe.

Another job of helper T cells is to alert killer T cells to join the battle. Killer T cells really do kill. Once activated and proliferated, they travel to the site of the infection, where they can recognize and destroy any antibody-decorated invader. They also can kill viruses that are inside cells, because the cells carry chemical signals that something has gone wrong inside. Tiny fragments of the invading viruses are displayed on the surface of a cell's membrane. Killer T cells recognize and bind with these fragments on infected cells and then signal the cells to commit suicide. The death of a cell kills the viruses inside it, too. However, killer T cells take time to activate and proliferate. Just like B cells, they take at least one week to proliferate and become killing machines.

Remembering the Enemy

Given time, the adaptive immune system can learn to mount a specific defense against any pathogen that causes disease, but the time lag can mean sickness and even increase the risk of death for an infected person. While Jeryl Lynn Hilleman lay sick with the mumps, however, her immune system responded just as it was supposed to respond. The mumps virus was recognized as foreign by her innate immune system. B cells and T cells proliferated. B cells made antibodies and tagged viruses for destruction; killer T cells destroyed any invaders that got inside cells. The virus did not escape to her brain or spinal cord. After about a week or two, the virus had been conquered. The swelling in Jeryl Lynn's lymph glands—where the virus attacked and B cells and T cells were proliferating—disappeared. Jeryl Lynn was well, and most of the B cells and T cells that had fought the conquered virus died out.

Jeryl Lynn's adaptive immune system, however, had one more important job. Not all of the B cells and T cells died out. Some of these experienced cells, still with the ability to recognize the mumps virus they had fought, became memory cells. It was these memory cells that gave Jeryl Lynn immunity to the mumps virus. She would be able to get the flu or catch a cold or come down with the measles, but should she ever again be exposed to the mumps virus, her memory cells would instantly recognize the invader and respond. There would be no lag time. T cells and B cells would proliferate so quickly that antibodies would decorate and opsonize the virus particles immediately, and then killer T cells, if needed, would join the fight with no delays. Sompayrac says, "As a result of this immunological memory, the adaptive system usually can spring into action so quickly during a second attack that you never even experience any symptoms."[6]

Vaccines Make Memories

Maurice Hilleman's mumps vaccine, just like every vaccine, would trigger immunological memory. And it would result in memory cells without the danger of actual sickness. Sompayrac compares vaccinations to war games:

> A vaccination is the immunological equivalent of the war games our armed forces use to prepare troops for battle. The goal of these "games" is to give soldiers as realistic a simulation of battle conditions as is possible without putting them in great danger. Likewise, a vaccination is intended to prepare the immune system for battle by giving the system as close a look at the real thing as is possible without exposing the vaccine recipient to undue risks. Consequently, the generals who plan war games and the scientists who develop vaccines have a common aim: maximum realism with minimum danger.[7]

In the case of the mumps virus, Hilleman accomplished "minimum danger" by making the virus helpless and weak. He grew the virus from his daughter's throat on the cells of chicken embryos (fertilized eggs) in his lab. Viruses grown from the same parent cell (for example, a mumps virus) but with varying characteristics (such as growing well in chickens instead of humans) are called strains. Hilleman named his mumps viruses grown in chicken cells the Jeryl Lynn strain. As the virus strain adapted to growing in chicken cells, the viruses became less and less adept at

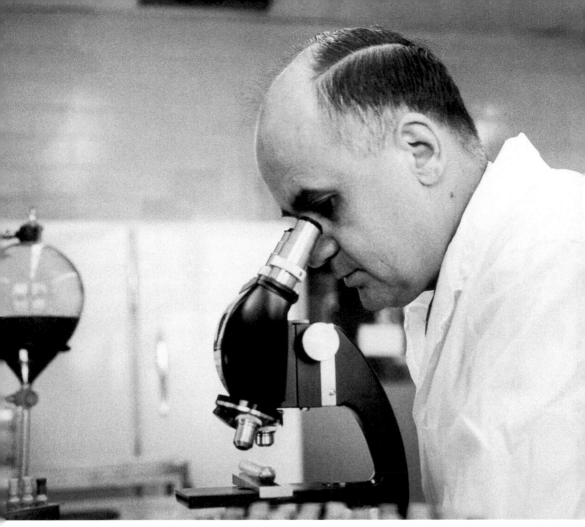

Maurice Hilleman checks a tissue culture for virus growth in 1963, the same year his daughter came down with mumps. Hilleman developed vaccines for several illnesses including mumps, measles, and hepatitis B.

growing in human cells. They changed as they got used to living in chicken cells. They became good at infecting chicken embryos but very poor at infecting humans. However, they maintained the "maximum realism" of the mumps virus. They still appeared to be foreign invaders to the innate immune system. They still presented the same antigens on their surfaces that triggered the proliferation of mumps antibodies. Some experienced T cells and B cells still became memory cells, ready to respond immediately should the virus ever attack again. When injected into a person, the vaccine conferred immunological memory for the mumps, even though that person never got sick.

Different Types of Vaccines

Immunological memory is the way all vaccines protect against disease, but scientists have developed different strategies to trigger that memory. Some vaccines, such as Hilleman's mumps vaccine, are attenuated vaccines. This means that the pathogens are alive but weakened and crippled. They are, for the most part, easy for the immune system to overcome and destroy. They trigger the production of memory cells that are primed and ready for a second attack. Other vaccines are made from pathogens that are killed. These pathogens—either viruses or bacteria— are grown in the lab and then destroyed, often with the disinfectant formaldehyde. Formaldehyde affects many pathogens by chemically gluing together the proteins that make up their cells. The pathogen still appears to be a live one to the immune system even though it is nonfunctional and cannot infect cells. When these dead pathogens are injected into people, they

attenuated

Weakened, but still able to cause an immune system response.

trigger an immune response that leads to the development of antibodies and memory cells.

Other vaccines are made by using only parts of pathogens and are called subunit vaccines. The vaccine for the bacteria that cause tetanus, for example, is not made of whole tetanus bacteria. It is made only of the toxins the bacteria produce. The toxins are weakened and then injected into people, where B cells react to the toxins by producing antibodies and memory cells. Some vaccines use only fragments of the bacterium's cell. The fragments may be, for example, the proteins of the cell wall that are antigens. These vaccines cannot possibly cause disease because the whole bacterium is not injected, but the antigens still trigger a strong antibody response. Such vaccines are known as acellular vaccines. The whooping cough vaccine is an acellular vaccine. Some viral vaccines are made of protein molecules stripped from the whole virus. The hepatitis B vaccine is made this way, and because it is not whole, it cannot cause infection, although it can cause an immune system response.

> **subunit vaccines**
>
> Vaccines made of proteins stripped from a pathogen so that the vaccines contain antigens but nothing that can infect human cells.

The Complex Problem of the Right Vaccine

When scientists set out to develop vaccines for infectious diseases, they do not face an easy task. They must figure out, often by trial and error, which strategy is best and how to make the vaccine effective without putting people in danger. Some killed pathogens do not trigger enough antibody production to protect against disease. Neither do some fragments of some pathogens. Some live pathogens, even when they are weakened, are too dangerous to inject into people and perhaps risk giving them the disease because, for example, just one virus in the vaccine is not weak enough. Other pathogens provoke an immune response that does not prevent disease when a person is exposed to the pathogen in the real world. Still other pathogens come in different varieties, all of which must be included in the vaccine for it to confer immunity. Some pathogens are difficult to "capture," meaning that they are hard to isolate and grow in the lab. Pathogens may carry so many different proteins on their surfaces that identifying the ones that are antigens is a huge problem. Some human viruses grow very poorly on lab animal cells. Each vaccine has to be tailored to the disease-causing pathogen.

Hilleman was able to surmount all the possible problems, and his Jeryl Lynn mumps vaccine was approved for use in the United States in 1967. One newspaper of the time summed up the vaccine's effectiveness by saying, "Jeryl recovered from mumps virus, but mumps virus never recovered from infecting Jeryl."[8] Hilleman's mumps vaccine is still used today and has almost eliminated mumps infections in many countries around the world. For many other deadly diseases, however, vaccines are still a work in progress.

Vaccines and Viruses

Maurice Hilleman successfully developed nine vaccines that are still used today, including vaccines for measles, rubella, hepatitis A, and hepatitis B, but he failed in his efforts to prevent the common cold. When Hilleman collected samples from people during the 1960s, he discovered why a vaccine was not possible. With his samples, he identified 54 different kinds of viruses that caused colds. (Today more than 100 different cold viruses are known.) Hilleman remarked, "If there was just one type, then a vaccine could protect against colds for the rest of your life: just like the measles and mumps vaccines."[9] However, the virus types are so varied that antibodies produced in response to one strain of cold virus do not recognize other kinds and so cannot confer immunity. Hilleman searched for similarities among his many cold viruses but finally concluded, "There was just no crossing at all between these strains."[10]

The Nature of Viruses

Modern vaccine researchers face the same problem that Hilleman did with cold viruses. There are too many virus types for a vaccine to be practical. Rhinoviruses (the viruses that cause about half of all colds) are a good example of why viral vaccine development can be complex. The basic nature of viruses can be extremely variable: Some easily develop new strains; some are specialized while others are flexible; and some have developed strategies that can evade and trick the immune system. Nevertheless, all viruses cause infection in a generally similar way—they attack cells.

Viruses are extremely tiny packages of genetic material, enclosed within a protein shell called a capsid. Typical viruses range from about 17 to 300 nanometers long. (One nanometer equals one billionth of a meter. For comparison, the diameter of a human hair is about 50,000 nanometers.) The proteins of its shell determine which kinds of cells a virus can infect. In the presence of a compatible cell, the virus latches on to the cell wall and then slips inside. Common cold viruses, for example, can bind only to the cells of the human upper respiratory tract.

Hijacking Cell Coding

Once inside cells, says science writer Corey Binns, viruses act on the cells by "turning them into virus Xerox machines."[11] Viruses cannot reproduce on their own; they can only do this in living cells. Binns explains:

capsid
The protein shell that surrounds a virus.

"A virus does contain some genetic information critical for making copies of itself, but it can't get the job done without the help of a cell's duplicating equipment, borrowing enzymes and other molecules to concoct more virus."[12] The virus uses its own genetic instructions to direct the living cell to make more viruses. The genetic instructions enclosed within the capsid are nucleic acid, either deoxyribonucleic acid (DNA) or ribonucleic acid (RNA). DNA carries coding instructions for living things, while RNA carries a kind of decoded copy of DNA instructions. RNA viruses mimic the messages carried in the living cell they infect. DNA viruses, which are more common, substitute their own DNA codes for the cell's DNA coding.

Viruses inside cells lose their capsids and then inject their own genetic material into the cell. In a complex series of steps, the factory of the cell begins to use the nucleic acid instructions to form new viruses. Then the many cell-manufactured viruses burst or leak from the cell and go on to infect more cells. Over and over, infecting viruses instruct cells, "Start making viruses." Some viruses need only 24 minutes to complete the process, explode out of a cell, and begin to infect and destroy more cells.

mutations
Permanent changes in DNA or genetic material that alter coded information and heredity.

Variable Viruses

Whenever viruses replicate, the nucleic acids must be copied, and sometimes mistakes, or mutations, occur that are like typographical errors in the coding instructions. RNA viruses in particular can have a very high mutation rate, which may change their antigens enough that the immune system does not recognize the new pathogen. Rhinoviruses, for example, are RNA viruses that typically make one copying error each time they replicate, so mutated strains develop very easily.

How Viruses Infect the Body

Viruses, which can enter the body through the nose, mouth, or breaks in the skin or membranes, are microscopic fragments of nucleic acid that are enclosed in protein shells. Viruses cannot reproduce on their own; instead, they must invade living "host" cells and use the cells as factories where they produce more viral material, and in this way they lead to various types of infection. This illustration shows the progression.

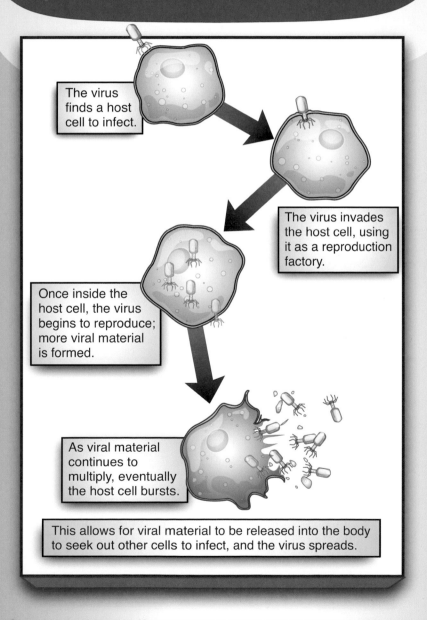

The virus finds a host cell to infect.

The virus invades the host cell, using it as a reproduction factory.

Once inside the host cell, the virus begins to reproduce; more viral material is formed.

As viral material continues to multiply, eventually the host cell bursts.

This allows for viral material to be released into the body to seek out other cells to infect, and the virus spreads.

Source: Craig Freudenrich, "How Viruses Work," How Stuff Works, 2000. http://health.howstuffworks.com.

DNA viruses are relatively stable. Smallpox, for instance, is a DNA virus that mutates slowly and for which a vaccine was so effective that smallpox has been exterminated. Mutation rates often determine whether or not researchers can develop effective vaccines against viral diseases. How specific a virus is to certain kinds of cells is important, too. Smallpox was specific to human hosts and thus, once eradicated from humans, died out completely. A virus that is able to grow in several different kinds of animals, such as the influenza virus, has other hosts from which to reinfect humans and is much harder to eradicate. However, viruses that grow only in humans may be a problem for vaccine researchers. What cells will they use in the laboratory to capture and grow their viruses in order to develop a vaccine?

Nancy Cox: Virologist

Since her college days, Iowa native Nancy Cox has been researching influenza viruses and how the virus infects its hosts. She has a doctorate in virology from the University of Cambridge in England. Cox is the chief of the Centers for Disease Control and Prevention's (CDC) Influenza Division, and it was her responsibility to shape the CDC's response to the threat of a 2009 H1N1 flu pandemic. In 2006 she had researched the possibility of a pandemic with bird flu. Bird flu does not travel easily among people. However, Cox worried that the virus could mutate and become a highly infectious strain as it exchanged DNA with regular flu viruses. Under carefully controlled conditions, she combined the virus with a flu virus that is highly contagious in people and worked to develop a vaccine. Her virus strain mutated so quickly that a single vaccine could not protect against it.

When strains of the new 2009 H1N1 virus were sent to the CDC for analysis, Cox thought her fears about a lethal flu virus mutation might be realized, but it was with a swine flu virus, not a bird flu virus. She and her research team analyzed the virus and provided the necessary information to the pharmaceutical companies that could rush development of a new vaccine. Fortunately, the 2009 H1N1 strain was not as lethal as she feared, but Cox has not become complacent about the dangers of a pandemic. She continues to monitor flu virus strains in her job as a guardian of the public health.

The Chickenpox Vaccine

Chickenpox is caused by the varicella virus and was once a common childhood disease. Typically, symptoms include an itchy rash of blisters on the skin, fever, headache, and sore throat. Usually, healthy children recover from the disease with no problems, but it can be more serious in teens and adults. Rarely, chickenpox can cause pneumonia, encephalitis (an inflammation in the brain), nerve damage, and vision loss. Babies are at greater risk of birth defects when their mothers get chickenpox during pregnancy. In the United States about 100 people died of chickenpox each year before there was a vaccine.

> **nucleic acid**
>
> A complex chemical compound in living cells or viruses that controls preservation, replication, and function.

Scientists wanted to be able to prevent chickenpox, but the varicella virus grows best in human cells. This was a major problem for vaccine researchers because varicella did not replicate well in chicken embryos. During the 1970s Japanese microbiologist Michiaki Takahashi began experimenting with the varicella virus. He knew he wanted to develop a live vaccine because live viruses provoke the best antibody response. He explained, "Since I knew that live vaccines induced solid immunity against diseases such as measles and polio, my thought from the beginning of the study was to develop a live attenuated varicella vaccine."[13] He collected the pus from a blister of a three-year-old boy infected with chickenpox. His next step was to grow it in the laboratory and attenuate it, but isolating the virus in a lab growth medium was difficult.

The answer came from the work of Leonard Hayflick and Stanley Plotkin in the United States during the 1960s. Hayflick had acquired cells from an aborted fetus in Sweden and had learned how to keep the cells frozen, alive, and able to replicate when thawed. Plotkin had used some of Hayflick's fetal cells to grow rubella viruses to develop a rubella vaccine. Hayflick once explained, "Every known human virus was found to grow in [human fetal cells]. That's what made them so attractive for vaccines."[14]

So Takahashi turned to human fetal cells for varicella. Over and over—11 different times—he grew his batch of varicella in successive dishes of fetal cells, lowering the temperature so that the viruses became progressively weaker. His varicella, forced to mutate slowly and adapt to growing at a temperature below 98.6°F (37°C), became less able to grow at normal human body temperature. Takahashi found that the virus would now grow in fetal cells from guinea pigs. So he grew, or passed, the viruses 12 more times in guinea pig fetal cells, weakening them still further. Then he replicated them by passing them twice through one set of human fetal cells and 5 times through another. The new strain of varicella was very weakened but alive. Unlike the natural varicella virus, it replicated very slowly. As the Vaccine Education Center of the Children's Hospital of Philadelphia explains, "Whereas natural viruses reproduce themselves thousands of times, vaccine viruses usually reproduce themselves fewer than 20 times."[15] Takahashi named his attenuated, slow-growing varicella the Oka strain, after the last name of the boy whose blister he had used for his sample virus.

At Merck, Hilleman used the Oka strain to develop a chickenpox vaccine in the United States. The strain was grown and multiplied in the laboratory and then purified. As is still done today, the resultant vaccine was combined with a fluid to carry the vaccine into the body. It was named Varivax, tested for safety, and introduced in the United States in 1995. By 2005 the incidence of chickenpox in the country had declined by 90 percent.

Objections to Using Human Fetal Cells

Today several vaccines are developed using human fetal cells, including those for rubella and hepatitis A, and this growth medium has been the source of some controversy. For vaccine makers, human fetal cells are ideal for growing any viruses that infect humans. Some people, however, view this choice as gravely immoral because the cells come from aborted fetuses, and they view abortion as the killing of potential human life. Debi Vinnedge is president and executive director of the pro-life organization Children of God for Life. She argues, "The fact is that casually accepting the use of aborted fetal cell lines in medical treatments has been a blatant disgrace to humanity, a despicable sullying of the value and dignity of human life and has leant credibility to the gross commercialization of aborted babies, ripped from their mothers' wombs—so that someone could turn a profit."[16] She believes that vaccines should be redeveloped without the use of human fetal cells and condemns pharmaceutical companies for not doing so. Many antiabortion groups agree with Vinnedge and worry that the use of fetal cells to develop vaccines will encourage future abortions. They argue that current technology now makes it possible to remake the vaccines in question using animal cells.

☢ An Outbreak of Mumps

In New York City in 2010, an outbreak of mumps sickened more than 1,500 people, most of them young Orthodox Jews, living in a close, religious community. Centers for Disease Control and Prevention (CDC) researchers discovered that the outbreak began at a boys' summer camp during June 2009. They reported that the initial U.S. infection started with 1 boy who had been infected with the virus during a visit to England, where many people fear the MMR (measles, mumps, rubella) vaccine and do not get their children vaccinated. Because of this, in 2009 England reported about 7,400 cases of mumps, as compared with about 300 in the United States.

Most of the U.S. mumps patients had been vaccinated. The CDC reported that 75 percent had received the 2 recommended doses. Two doses of the vaccine are believed to be 79 to 95 percent effective at providing immunity to mumps. However, no vaccine is 100 percent effective; immune system memory cells may be lost over time or may not be amply triggered in all people. The CDC also theorizes that prolonged or repeated exposure to the virus may trigger active infection better than a single exposure. Nevertheless, the outbreak did not spread to the wider community of New York City. No epidemic occurred, and most vaccinated people were protected. The CDC states, "Although vaccination alone does not prevent all mumps outbreaks, maintaining high measles, mumps, and rubella (MMR) vaccination coverage remains the most effective way to prevent outbreaks and limit their size when they occur."

Centers for Disease Control and Prevention, "Update: Mumps Outbreak—New York and New Jersey, June 2009–January 2010," Morbidity and Mortality Weekly Report, February 12, 2010. www.cdc.gov.

Modern researchers could redevelop vaccines without the use of human fetal cells, but the process would not be an easy or straightforward one. Finding appropriate animal cells, attenuating the viruses, and ensuring the safety and effectiveness of the vaccine would be a long, difficult, expensive task. The National Network for Immunization Information (NNii), a nonprofit, science-based organization, argues that currently it is neither feasible nor necessary to provide alternative vaccines to those made with aborted human cells. Only two cell lines are used to grow viruses for vaccines, and they have been in use for decades. One is from an abortion in the United States in 1961, labeled WI-38; the other is from a 1966 abortion in the United Kingdom, labeled MRC-5. Neither abortion had anything to do with developing vaccines. In addition, no new abortions are needed to produce any vaccines. The National Network for Immunization Information says, "The fetal tissues that eventually became WI-38 and the MRC-5 cell cultures were removed from fetuses that were dead. The cellular biologists who made the cell cultures did not induce the abortions."[17] These fetal cells are expected to provide the growth medium for vaccine production for generations to come.

A Cancer Vaccine

Not all of today's vaccines depend upon growing viruses in animal or human cells. In 2006 the human papillomavirus (HPV) vaccine was approved in the United States. This vaccine prevents the sexually transmitted HPV infection in women, which is the main cause of cervical cancer. In the United States about 10,000 women are diagnosed with cervical cancer each year, and approximately 3,700 die. HPV infection does not lead to cervical cancer in most women, but about 5 percent develop cancerous cells and then face a difficult course of treatment. On the Web site of the National Cervical Cancer Coalition, for example, Mrs. R. (real name withheld for her privacy) describes her battle with cervical cancer. She was diagnosed with the cancer at age 30 and had to undergo surgery to remove her uterus, ovaries, cervix, and nearby lymph nodes. Then she received 7 weeks of chemotherapy treatment and 28 radiation treatments to kill any possible surviving cancer cells. It was a frightening time for Mrs. R., but she was fortunate. In 2010, 4 years after her treatment began, she was still cancer free. In developing countries, cervical cancer treatment is not readily available as it was for Mrs. R.; about half the women who are diagnosed with cervical cancer each year in developing countries die.

To prevent cervical cancer by preventing HPV infection, researchers developed a new kind of vaccine using knowledge about the gene that codes for the papillomavirus's protein shell. Over a period of 15 years, researchers from four different laboratories in the United States and Australia contributed to the vaccine's development before it was introduced by the pharmaceutical companies Merck and GlaxoSmithKline.

The HPV vaccine is a subunit vaccine made through genetic engineering. First the researchers isolated the gene in HPV that codes for the protein shell. This gene was then inserted into the genetic coding of single-celled microorganisms, either insect cells or yeasts. The cells incorporated the coding into their own genetic coding and began producing the protein. Scientist Jacqueline Jaeger Houtman says, "Those cells could then crank out viral proteins," and when they did,

A young woman is vaccinated against HPV, the virus that causes cervical cancer. About 10,000 women are diagnosed with cervical cancer annually in the United States, where deaths from the disease total about 3,700 each year.

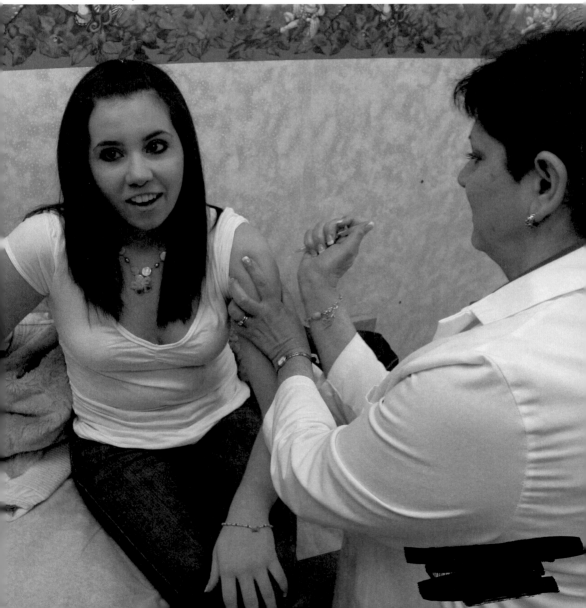

"something interesting happened."[18] The proteins spontaneously re-arranged themselves into a whole virus shell, called a virus-like particle (VLP). Houtman explains: "It contained no DNA, so it could not multiply or cause cancer. VLPs looked just like the real virus under the electron microscope. They could fool the eye, but could they fool the immune system?"[19]

> ### virus-like particle
>
> The proteins of a virus shell that have self-assembled into a spherical capsid that does not contain genetic material but can cause an immune system response.

They could and did. The antigens of the protein shell provoked a strong antibody response. The only trouble was that the antibodies protected only against the particular type of HPV from which the VLPs were derived. Therefore, Gardasil, the vaccine produced by Merck and made with yeasts, contains VLPs derived from 4 different HPV types—2 types that cause 70 percent of all cervical cancers, and 2 types that cause genital warts. In 2009 this vaccine also was approved for males to prevent the infection of their sexual partners and to prevent genital warts. GlaxoSmith-Kline's vaccine, called Cervarix, is produced in insect cells and contains only VLPs for the 2 HPV types that cause cervical cancer. The vaccines are not completely effective because at least 13 other types of HPV cause about 30 percent of cervical cancers. As yet, no vaccine can prevent these types, nor can the vaccines help people who are already infected with HPV. Nevertheless, since 250,000 women worldwide die from cervical cancer every year, thousands of lives could be saved with the HPV vaccines. Says Robert Rose, a codeveloper at the University of Rochester, "It's been an amazing life experience. It's been thrilling—that what we've done could affect the world."[20]

Influenza Vaccines

Someday many viral vaccines may be made using VLPs. They have the advantage of replicating quickly and yet carrying no genetic coding for infection. For these reasons vaccines made with VLPs are particularly attractive to researchers working on flu vaccines. Influenza viruses continually mutate into new strains, are flexible enough to infect animals as well as humans, and can even swap genetic material with each other inside cells to create completely new types of viruses. The most important antigens on the surfaces of flu viruses give the strains their names. The first are called hemagglutinins. There are 16 types of hemagglutinins, which change slightly every year. The other major flu virus antigen is called neuraminidase, and it also changes so that different types of flu viruses evolve. Two types—N1 and N2—are responsible for human flu infections. Antibodies that protect against one type of flu cannot protect against the other types. That is why flu vaccines must be redeveloped every year, as flu season begins. The viruses have changed since the previous year's vaccine was made. It is because of this constant mutation that medical doctor and vaccine developer Paul A. Offit says, "Pandemics of influenza are inevitable."[21]

Pandemics are what vaccine researchers and public health officials fear most when they work to develop yearly flu vaccines. Three types of hemagglutinins have caused all of the human flu pandemics known throughout history. They are labeled H1, H2, and H3. Worldwide flu pandemics occur when a virus has changed so much that few people have antibodies to protect them and when vaccine developers have been unsuccessful at predicting which type of flu is likely. This situation is what scientists feared in April 2009 when a new strain of flu virus was detected—one now called 2009 H1N1. Although H1N1 had been identified in 1986 in Taiwan, its genetic material had changed just enough that few people around the world had any antibodies against it.

2009 H1N1

Development of yearly flu vaccines begins each year in February, when scientists try to predict which flu viruses will be the most likely to infect people during the next flu season. By the time flu season rolls around, they have produced ample amounts of attenuated or killed flu viruses and millions of doses of vaccines. Production is accomplished in the traditional way—by growing the viruses in chicken embryos. When 2009 H1N1 was identified, the seasonal flu vaccine for 2009 was already in production to prevent three types of flu strains—an H1N1 strain, an H3N2 strain, and a different kind of virus named influenza B. The seasonal flu vaccine could not protect anyone from 2009 H1N1, but a vaccine could not be made until the specific antigens were isolated, analyzed, and identified.

At the CDC, researchers worked feverishly to figure out if the new flu viruses that had already infected people were structured in the same way or had multiple new antigens. By the end of May, they knew that they were dealing with 50 different 2009 H1N1 strains, but that all the new strains had similar antigens. Only one vaccine would be necessary, so the CDC sent the isolated viruses to vaccine manufacturers to be grown in fertilized eggs. Nancy Cox, the director of the CDC's flu division, worried that a flu pandemic was possible. She said, "It is very clear to us that flu virus can cause serious illness and death. This pandemic virus is no exception. It is very clear a vaccine should be developed."[22] She and other scientists hoped that 100 million doses of a vaccine against 2009 H1N1 could be developed for the United States by the time flu season began in the fall. However, vaccine makers need about six months to produce flu vaccines. Wellington Sun of the U.S. Food and Drug Administration (FDA) commented, "Time is really not on our side."[23]

A factory worker in China checks eggs used for growing influenza virus for an H1N1 vaccine. Approximately 1.2 billion fertilized chicken eggs were needed for the production of 3 billion doses of flu vaccine to be distributed worldwide in 2009.

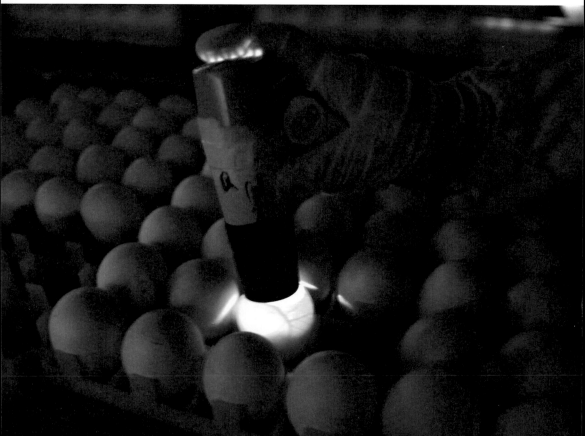

For vaccinations worldwide, 3 billion doses of the flu vaccine were needed. To manufacture this much vaccine requires approximately 1.2 billion fertilized chicken eggs. Even though whole chicken farms are devoted to supplying eggs for vaccine makers, acquiring so many eggs takes time. Then each egg must be injected with the virus, which must be grown for about 3 days. Next the virus has to be attenuated or killed and then purified, so that the antigens are available to make the vaccine. Altogether, the process takes about 2 weeks for each batch of vaccine in each egg—if the virus grows as rapidly as expected. Unlike the viruses that cause seasonal flu, however, 2009 H1N1 did not replicate as well as expected. The batches from each egg were 5 to 10 times smaller than batches from other flu strains. This complication meant that vaccine makers failed to get an ample supply of H1N1 vaccine to the public before the flu season started in the fall.

Toward a Better Vaccine

Richard Compans, a vaccine expert at Emory University in Georgia, says of the months it takes to produce a vaccine, "Use of chicken eggs is [a] kind of old-fashioned and time-consuming procedure."[24] This is why he and other modern researchers want to develop a VLP vaccine for 2009 H1N1. Compans explains, "You could cut out several months, get it down to at least on the order of as little as two months."[25] A VLP vaccine for 2009 H1N1 was developed by a biotechnology company called Novavax, but it was still being tested for safety and effectiveness during the 2009–2010 flu season. Cox predicts that the effort to create this new flu vaccine will not be wasted. In February 2010 she warned, "We expect the 2009 H1N1 virus to be around for a long time."[26] Vaccine researchers are in an almost constant battle to stay one step ahead of the changeable viruses that cause disease.

Vaccines and Bacteria

I n March 2009 one-month-old Dana McCaffery of New South Wales, Australia, died from whooping cough, also known as pertussis. Her symptoms began mildly, with a runny nose and a cough, but very quickly the infant became severely ill and had to be hospitalized. Her parents remember:

> There is no treatment to cure Whooping Cough and we had to watch in horror as the Pertussis took its course. . . . First, our tiny daughter coughed uncontrollably. . . . Dana developed Pneumonia on the third day. . . . On the fifth day, the Pertussis took an unexpected and deadly turn. In what seemed an instant, Dana had an aggressive reaction to the toxin, which attacked her immune system and heart. The Pertussis blocked every drug or treatment that the team of specialists could throw at it. We were powerless to save her. After nearly 10 hours of desperate blood transfusions, Dana's beautiful heart stopped beating and she let out her last sweet breath.[27]

Dangerous Bacteria

The toxin to which the McCafferys refer is the poison released by the *Bordetella pertussis* bacterium that causes whooping cough. Bacteria that produce toxins are especially deadly when they infect young children, although most teens and adults recover from whooping cough without problems. A pertussis vaccine was developed in 1926, but Dana was still too young to be vaccinated when she was apparently infected by an un-vaccinated person who carried the bacterium and sneezed or coughed, sending the germ through the air and into Dana's airways. Dana's death was a rarity in Australia, where most children are vaccinated, but whooping cough remains a serious danger today for unvaccinated children. In 2001, for example, 340,000 children died of the disease in the developing world. Bacterial infections are often much more dangerous than viral infections. They also are often much more difficult to prevent by means of a vaccine. As pathogens, bacteria are very different from viruses.

Long before scientists knew what viruses were, they saw and identified bacteria. Bacteria are very small—a typical bacterium is between 1 and 5 micrometers in size (a micrometer is one-millionth of a meter)—and must be magnified 1,000 times to be seen under a microscope. However, the smallest bacterium is larger than the biggest virus. Viruses can be seen

The rod-shaped Bordetella pertussis *bacteria (yellow) that cause whooping cough are shown in this scanning electron micrograph of a section of tracheal tissue. A vaccine for whooping cough, also known as pertussis, was developed in 1926.*

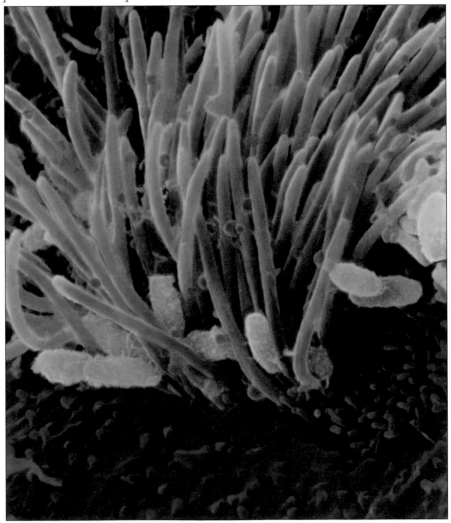

only through electron microscopes that magnify them 1 million times. Yet vaccines for viral diseases were developed before viruses were ever seen and about 100 years before the first bacterial vaccine was developed. In part, it took so much longer for researchers to make bacterial vaccines because bacteria are more complicated than viruses. Today some bacterial vaccines are similar to viral vaccines, but others require different strategies and are made in unique ways.

Bacteria and the Immune System

A typical bacterium is a single cell surrounded by a hard capsule or shell. Inside the cell's membrane is the bacterium's genetic material, arranged as a single, long chain of DNA. Unlike viruses, bacteria are able to survive on their own. They can live, for example, in dust, on a table, on the surface of human skin, or in a water pipe—anywhere that they can find a favorable environment and enough food (such as sugar or proteins) to survive and reproduce. Bacteria reproduce by cell division. One bacterium becomes 2, then 4, and so on, and given enough food, can become a colony of millions or even billions of bacteria in the space of a few hours. In 1 gram (0.035 ounce) of soil, for example, there could be 2.5 billion bacteria. When pathogenic bacteria are able to break through the barriers of the human skin and mucous membranes, they can grow and reproduce just as rapidly within the environment of the human body and the bloodstream.

Just like viruses, bacteria have surface antigens made of proteins that can be recognized by the immune system and can trigger antibody production. However, bacteria have many more proteins than simple viruses. Paul A. Offit explains, "For example, measles virus contains ten proteins, and mumps virus contains nine. Bacteria are much larger; pneumococcus [the pneumonia-causing bacterium] contains about two thousand proteins."[28]

encapsulated

Enclosed in a capsule or protective shell.

Figuring out which of all these proteins are the antigens complicates the development of bacterial vaccines, as does the protective capsule that surrounds many pathogenic bacteria. The bacteria that cause pneumonia, typhoid, meningitis, and streptococcus infections, for example, are known as encapsulated bacteria because of the protective capsule. Commonly, this capsule is made of thick complex sugars called

According to the Centers for Disease Control and Prevention, any vaccine can cause side effects. In most cases doctors and medical researchers determine that the risks of the disease are greater than the risks of any vaccine side effects for the vast majority of the population. Usually vaccine reactions are mild; they may include soreness or redness at the injection site or low fever that passes quickly. Rarely, a severe reaction may occur. For example, the DTaP (diphtheria, tetanus, and acellular pertussis) vaccine has been reported to cause a severe allergic reaction in 1 out of 1 million vaccinated children. This reaction may include coma, seizures, or permanent brain damage. Researchers are not positive that these reactions are due to vaccination, because reports of them are so rare, but they are considered possible reactions.

Because several vaccines are grown in eggs, they can be dangerous for anyone with a serious egg allergy, and these vaccines are not recommended for egg-allergic people. Their immune systems mount an overwhelming response to the egg proteins. The reaction usually occurs within a few minutes after injection and can be life threatening. People may also have an allergic reaction to the preservatives and other chemicals added to vaccines. Although usually not life threatening, the vaccine may make these people ill.

polysaccharides, and it sometimes covers and hides the antigens from the immune system. To make matters worse, bacteria are also as capable of rapidly mutating and tricking the immune system as are viruses.

Vaccines from Whole Bacteria

Once introduced into the human body, bacteria can be hardy, extremely dangerous, and sometimes lethal. For this reason, developing safe vaccines with whole, attenuated bacteria has been very difficult. If even one bacterium maintains the ability to grow and reproduce, the result could be disastrous since the vaccine would actually give the person the disease. Some of the first bacterial vaccines were made of whole, killed bacteria. For example, a vaccine against the bacterium *Salmonella typhi*, which causes typhoid fever, was developed in 1896 by English scientist Almroth Wright. Typhoid fever causes high fever, abdominal pain, intestinal ruptures, and hemorrhages, as well as symptoms such as unconsciousness, delirium, and psychosis. About 10 percent of untreated individuals die, and in developing countries, typhoid kills about 200,000 people each year. Thousands of others are left with permanent disabilities. At the time Wright was working, typhoid fever killed up to 30 percent of its victims because there were no antibiotics. Wright developed his vaccine by isolating the bacteria and killing them with heat. This approach worked because many pathogenic bacteria require a temperature range similar to that of the human body in order to survive. (The immune system generates a fever for the same reason: to kill the infecting bacteria.)

Whole, killed vaccines are called inactivated vaccines and have saved thousands of lives, but they do not trigger as strong an immune response as do live vaccines. Because the bacteria are dead, they do not replicate at all and, therefore, are cleared from the body so quickly that a complete immune system response is not activated. This means that enough long-lasting memory cells are not produced, immunity wears off over time, and booster shots are required periodically. Whole killed bacterial vaccines also can cause side effects. Since every antigen is still present on the whole bacterial cells, these killed vaccines do cause a temporarily strong initial response that often leads to inflammation, soreness at the injection site, and fever. Nevertheless, because killed bacterial vaccines are generally safe, one kind of typhoid vaccine used today continues to be a whole, killed vaccine.

Instead of Whole Bacteria

Some bacteria are dangerous not because of their multiplication in the human body but because they produce toxins. The toxins of diphtheria and tetanus bacteria can be as deadly as pertussis toxins. Tetanus is especially dangerous and kills 25 percent of infected, untreated people. Once introduced into the body, usually through a wound or injury, the bacterium multiplies and produces a poison called tetanospasmin. This toxin attacks the nerve cells in the human spinal cord and causes muscle spasms that are so strong that they can tear muscles and fracture the spine. Breathing muscles can be paralyzed.

Early in the twentieth century, researchers discovered that killed toxins, called toxoids, could generate the production of antibodies and confer immunity. The toxins are isolated in the lab, killed with formaldehyde, and purified. Vaccines for diphtheria and tetanus are still made from toxoids today and are safe because the bacteria themselves form no part of the vaccines; only inactivated toxins are required. For both diphtheria and tetanus, however, memory cells must be refreshed with booster shots (so called because they "boost" protection), and temporary side effects are still possible.

toxoids

Inactivated or altered bacterial toxins in which the toxic properties are destroyed but retain the ability to trigger antibodies and an immune system response.

Inactivated bacterial vaccines continue to be the choice of researchers today, but modern developers rely on parts of bacteria instead of whole bacteria to make subunit vaccines that are safe and effective. The pertussis vaccine in current use was introduced in the United States in 1991. It is made not of whole killed bacteria but the inactivated toxins and antigens that can trigger an immune response. It is referred to as an acellular vaccine and is considered to be safer, cause fewer side effects, and be just as effective as the old inactivated vaccine.

Volunteers are vaccinated against typhoid fever at the U.S. Army Medical School in Washington, D.C. Although the vaccine was developed in 1896, it is unavailable in many developing countries, where typhoid still kills or maims thousands of people each year.

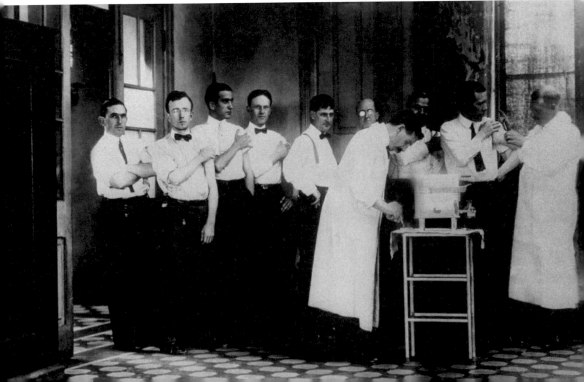

Polysaccharide Vaccines

The polysaccharides that form the capsule that surrounds pneumococcus—the bacterium that causes pneumonia—are also used to develop vaccines. Untreated bacterial pneumonia can kill 30 percent of its victims when it infects the lungs, and even with treatment, it can kill people weakened with other diseases. Former president Ronald Reagan, for example, weakened with Alzheimer's disease, died of pneumonia. For researchers, the difficulty in creating a pneumonia vaccine lay in the fact that there are at least 90 different strains of pneumococci. During the 1940s researchers discovered how to strip the polysaccharide shell from bacteria and learned that this capsule alone generated the formation of antibodies. However, the antibodies that protected against one strain of pneumococcus were useless against other strains.

During the 1960s and 1970s, U.S. doctor Robert Austrian determined that just 14 strains caused 80 percent of the pneumococcus infections in people. He made a vaccine that contained the polysaccharides from the 14 strains and tested his vaccine on gold miners in South Africa, who had a high incidence of bacterial pneumonia because of their working conditions. The vaccine worked and reduced the incidence of pneumonia in the miners by 80 percent, but in the developed world, no one was interested in a pneumonia vaccine.

> **polysaccharides**
>
> Complex carbohydrate structures made up of multiple sugar molecules.

Since antibiotics worked so well to cure pneumonia, most scientists and doctors believed a vaccine was unnecessary. Austrian had researched the rates of death from pneumonia in the United States, however, and demonstrated that many of the elderly and the very young died quickly of pneumonia despite antibiotic treatment. He insisted that prevention would save thousands of lives. No one would listen except Maurice Hilleman, who persuaded Merck to produce the vaccine. By 1983 Hilleman and Austrian developed a pneumonia vaccine that contained more capsule polysaccharides from more strains. Austrian said, "This is probably the most complex vaccine that we have. It's designed to protect against twenty-three different infections."[29] By 1991 the pneumonia vaccine was recommended for all people 65 and older. One injection was all that was needed for immunity to the 23 kinds of pneumococcus that cause bacterial pneumonia.

When Treatment Fails

Antibiotic drugs kill bacteria and are the treatment of choice for bacterial infections such as pneumonia, meningitis, and tuberculosis. When antibiotics were new to the world in the 1940s, they killed bacteria easily, but that is no longer true. As antibiotics were used more and more, many bacteria gradually mutated into new strains that resist and survive antibiotic treatment. For example, all pneumococci used to be susceptible to penicillin. Today at least 25 percent of pneumococcus strains are resistant to penicillin.

Vaccines are the answer to the terrible problem of antibiotic-resistant bacteria, say experts, because they confer immunity to bacterial diseases and make treatment efforts unnecessary. Antibiotic resistance is one of the main reasons that a tuberculosis vaccine is urgently needed. The *Haemophilus influenzae* type B, or Hib, vaccine came just in time to make people immune to the antibiotic-resistant bacteria that cause meningitis. Since the vaccine's introduction in 1990, meningitis caused by both resistant and nonresistant Hib strains has been reduced by 99 percent in the United States. Pneumonia vaccines today actually protect against the pneumococcus strains most likely to become drug resistant. "Vaccines may eventually stand alone as our last chance to fight bacterial infections," says vaccine developer Paul A. Offit.

Paul A. Offit, *Vaccinated: One Man's Quest to Defeat the World's Deadliest Diseases.* New York: HarperCollins, 2008, p. 155.

Modern Conjugate Vaccines

The polysaccharide pneumonia vaccine, however, could not protect young children. Polysaccharides do not provoke an immune response and antibody generation in children under the age of about two and a half or three. Researchers do not yet completely understand why this is so, but they do know that infants are born with immature immune systems. Babies cannot make antibodies to polysaccharides. Without this antibody, T cells do not activate, and there can be no memory cells. Since polysaccharide encapsulated bacteria can cause severe meningitis and pneumonia, as well as ear and sinus infections, in young children, this was a major issue to vaccine researchers. The answer was introduced in the United States in 2000 and was a new kind of pneumonia vaccine called a conjugate vaccine.

A conjugate vaccine is one in which a weak antigen (the polysaccharides) is combined with a strong antigen in order to provoke a full immune response. Even infants can produce antibodies to some antigens. In the case of pneumococci, Ronald J. Eby of Wyeth Pharmaceuticals spent 15 years searching for the protein substance that infant immune systems could recognize and attack. In the laboratory he chemically linked a protein antigen to the polysaccharide shell of the bacterium. The protein was a toxin from the bacterium that causes diphtheria. The toxin is made harmless, but it is recognized by the immune system as a foreign invader and so, therefore, is the polysaccharide shell. It stimulates helper T cells and ensures the production of memory cells.

> ### conjugate vaccine
>
> A vaccine made by chemically bonding a poor antigen, such as a polysaccharide, with a protein that triggers a good immune system response.

Eby and his research team decided to make the vaccine for the 7 most common bacterial strains that caused about 80 percent of pneumococcus infection in North America. That meant 7 different polysaccharides that are linked to the protein, all combined into 1 vaccine. It was named Prevnar and introduced in the United States in 2000. By 2008 Prevnar had reduced the incidence of pneumococcus infection in children under 5 years old by 78 percent. The scientist in charge of testing Eby's vaccine, Dace V. Madore, said, "The possibility of saving lives is why all of us enjoy working in vaccines."[30]

More Polysaccharides for More Protection

By 2007 Prevnar had reduced by 99 percent the number of infections caused by the seven strains in the vaccine. However, it provided no protection for other pneumococcus strains. Different strains are more common in different parts of the world. In developing countries, such as in Africa, other strains still cause about 1 million deaths each year. Then in 2005, due to the overuse of antibiotics, a strain of pneumococcus mutated into an antibiotic-resistant form and could no longer be effectively treated. The incidence of pneumococcus infection began to rise.

A better vaccine was needed, and Wyeth researchers went back to work. In February 2010, Prevnar 13 was introduced to the world. The new vaccine is made in the same way as Prevnar but now protects against 13 types of pneumococci, including the antibiotic-resistant one. The World Health Organization (WHO) says that pneumococcal infections are the leading cause of preventable death in children under five years old throughout the world. Pfizer, the pharmaceutical company that bought Wyeth in 2009, is conducting global research with Prevnar 13 and promises to "collaborate with healthcare providers, governments, and local communities to support and expand access to reliable affordable healthcare around the world."[31]

Meningitis Vaccines

Prevnar was not the first conjugate vaccine to be developed to protect young children from deadly diseases. The Hib vaccine is a conjugate vaccine that protects against the *Haemophilus influenzae* type B bacterium that causes one kind of meningitis. Meningitis is an infection of the lining that surrounds the brain and spinal cord, and children who survive the disease often suffer nerve damage and permanent disability, such as mental retardation and epilepsy. Hib, too, is surrounded by a polysaccharide capsule that does not trigger an immune response in infants and toddlers. A conjugate vaccine had to be developed. The bacterial polysaccharides were linked with an antigen from a diphtheria toxin, and the vaccine for Hib was introduced in 1990. Since vaccination for Hib has become routine, the incidence of Hib infection has decreased by 99 percent throughout the developed world.

Another bacterium that causes meningitis is called *Neisseria meningitidis* and can be a problem for young people who live in close quarters such as in college dormitories. Although infection is relatively rare, it can have terrible consequences when it strikes. In 2005, for example, Ashley Lee, a college freshman at Indiana University, came down with this form of bacterial meningitis and became critically ill very quickly. *Neisseria meningitidis* is a disease affecting the spinal cord, its fluid, and the blood system. This meningitis type kills 10 to 12 percent of its victims despite medical treatment. The disease prevents normal blood flow, which can kill tissues and organs. Ashley survived her meningitis but not before doctors had to amputate one foot because it was dead from lack of blood flow. Other survivors of this kind of meningitis may be left with brain damage, hearing loss, or kidney disease.

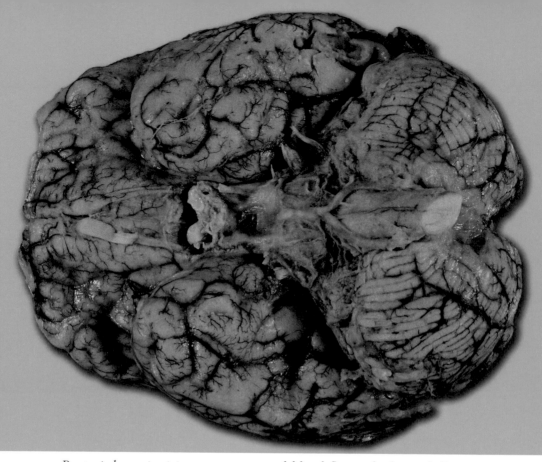

Bacterial meningitis prevents normal blood flow, which can kill tissues and organs. A brain specimen from a person who suffered from the disease shows signs of cell death, or necrosis, in the midbrain area.

Ironically, a conjugate vaccine that could have prevented Ashley's meningitis—Menactra—had been developed and introduced in that same year. Ashley's doctor did not have a supply and suggested that she get vaccinated at college. The busy student had not yet gotten around to it. She says, "I just didn't know the severity of it. I thought it was just, like, another vaccination."[32] Today the CDC recommends that all young people between the ages of 11 and 18 receive this lifesaving conjugate vaccine, and more than 30 states require that college students be informed about bacterial meningitis and the available vaccines. Many colleges require meningitis vaccinations for all incoming students.

Meningitis, however, remains far from conquered. Several kinds of viruses and bacteria (as well as other factors) can cause meningitis. In Asia and Africa a different kind of bacterium, known as type A, causes most cases of meningitis. Each year, the bacteria known as group A meningococci cause epidemics of meningitis in sub-Saharan Africa. The problem is so widespread that health officials have dubbed this part of Africa the "meningitis belt." Experts estimate that every year, 200,000 people get meningitis, and 1 in 10 infected children die. In Africa, up to 22 percent of survivors are left permanently deaf.

A Vaccine for Africa

There is no vaccine for group A bacteria. This situation is not due to lack of knowledge but to lack of funding. Vaccine makers have little demand for a group A vaccine in wealthy countries and therefore cannot afford the high cost of research and development needed to produce a vaccine. Sub-Saharan African countries are too poor to buy any expensive vaccines. In 2001 WHO and the nonprofit organization Program for Appropriate Technology in Health formed the Meningitis Vaccine Project (MVP) to address the need for a vaccine for Africa. Nigerian government official Hassane Adamou pleaded, "Please don't give us a vaccine we can't afford. That is worse than no vaccine."[33] The MVP estimated that the vaccine would have to cost no more than 50 cents per dose.

Two companies, one in Europe and the other in India, agreed to isolate and supply the polysaccharide shells and the tetanus toxoid needed to make the conjugate vaccine. A Maryland research lab agreed to develop the technology for conjugating the toxoid with the polysaccharide. Then the Indian company, Serum Institute of India, agreed to manufacture the vaccine for less than 50 cents a dose. By 2004 researchers at Serum Institute of India demonstrated that the vaccine, now named MenAfriVac, was safe and effective in animals, and testing in humans was begun in 2005. In January 2010 the MVP and Serum Institute of India began the final tests of the vaccine in India with 830 children between the ages of 5 and 10 years. The MVP predicts that the trials of MenAfriVac will be completed by 2012. If all goes well, the vaccine will then be ready for widespread distribution in Africa's meningitis belt.

The Last Step for Success

Developing a successful meningitis A vaccine is but the first step in protecting Africa's children. The MVP says, "Introducing the newly developed vaccine, making sure all at-risk children are protected, is our next big challenge."[34] The MVP plans a mass vaccination strategy, beginning in the African countries where meningitis epidemics are the worst and extending to countries with fewer yearly reported cases of meningitis. The first three countries where the vaccine will be distributed, in the heart of the meningitis belt, are Burkina Faso, Mali, and Niger. The MVP predicts that ample supplies of the conjugate vaccine will have to be produced for at least 10 years in order to protect whole populations in each country. "The definition of success," states the MVP Web site, "for the Meningitis Vaccine Project is the elimination of epidemic meningitis in sub-Saharan countries that introduce the meningococcal A conjugate vaccine."[35] For the vaccine producers and researchers who made the meningitis A vaccine, a safe and effective product is not enough—their ultimate goal is saving lives and ending the threat of meningitis epidemics in Africa.

Safe, Effective, and Approved

Bringing a new vaccine from the laboratory to general public use requires a process that can last for decades. Whatever the type of vaccine, researchers must determine that it does what it is supposed to do and will do no harm to the vast majority of the people who use it. These are not always easy determinations to make, and the decisions do not belong to the scientists alone. In the United States the FDA is the final authority for the approval of new drugs and vaccines. Researchers must prove to the federal government with extensive testing that their vaccine is effective and safe. Only then can they achieve governmental approval of the vaccine and offer it to the market. Ultimately, the success of any vaccine will depend on public acceptance, and here, too, researchers have an important role to play. Since no medicine or vaccine is 100 percent safe and effective, the risks must be balanced against the benefits.

Trial and Error

In the early days of vaccine development, researchers were quite limited in their ability to test their new vaccine preparations for safety and effectiveness. When Louis Pasteur developed the first rabies vaccine, he tested it by injecting the dried, ground-up spinal cords of rabbits infected with rabies into live, healthy dogs and rabbits. Fifteen days of drying killed the rabies virus, so the animals remained healthy. Over and over, Pasteur injected rabies-infected spinal cords that had been dried for fewer and fewer days. Then, on the last day, he injected live rabies preparations into the dogs and rabbits and waited to see if they died of rabies. They did not, and when nine-year-old Joseph Meister came to see Pasteur on July 6, 1885, the scientist simply made the decision to try the vaccine on a person and see if it worked.

The boy had been attacked by a rabid dog on July 4 and faced certain death without Pasteur's experimental vaccine. There was no medical treatment for rabies, and it is almost always fatal. Pasteur had no way of knowing whether the injections would kill Joseph; up to this point he had only experimented on dogs and rabbits. After beginning the injections, Pasteur wrote to his children, "I cannot come to terms with the idea of applying a measure of last resort to this child. And yet [I have] to go through with it. The little fellow continues to feel very well."[36] Twelve times more, Pasteur injected Joseph with material that was less and less dried. This meant that Joseph was receiving killed viruses, then attenuated viruses, then live viruses. The boy did not die but became the first person ever to survive the bite of an animal with rabies.

Pasteur's vaccine worked, even though Joseph had already been exposed to rabies, because it overcame the virus's ability to trick the immune system. Instead of traveling through the bloodstream, where the immune system would discover it, the rabies virus travels through the nerves to reach the spinal cord and brain. Vaccination puts the virus directly into the bloodstream, where it is recognized by the immune system, and plentiful antibody production prevents infection before the slow moving virus reaches the spinal cord.

The Importance of Animals Today

With no other means available to him at the time, Pasteur had relied entirely on a relatively brief period of animal testing of his rabies vaccine. This would not happen today. Even the most basic vaccines take years of testing before they receive approval for use in humans. Vaccine development now is a multistep, regulated process with layers of safety checks. Despite these changes, modern vaccine developers still use animal testing for a preliminary determination of a vaccine's effectiveness and safety. They draw blood from the animals to check for immune responses and measure the number of antibodies made in response to the vaccination. They inject the animals with the disease-causing bacteria and viruses and then determine how quickly and efficiently the pathogens are removed by the immune system. They evaluate the animals' health to be sure that the new vaccine does not, for instance, raise blood pressure, cause liver damage, or lead to birth defects.

Animal testing is the first step in the process of bringing a vaccine to the public. In many countries around the world, national governments require extensive animal testing before any new drug or vaccine can be approved for testing in humans. In the United States researchers and pharmaceutical companies must provide proof to the FDA that animal

⚛ A Human-Made Disaster

When Jonas Salk developed the first polio vaccine, he used a thick asbestos filter to separate the viruses from the bits of dead cells left over from growing them and killed the viruses with formaldehyde. The filtering made the vaccine pure and safe. Clinical trials in 1954 proved that the vaccine was effective and triggered antibody production. In 1955, 5 U.S. pharmaceutical companies began to manufacture the vaccine in large quantities. One of them, however, named Cutter Laboratories, made a terrible manufacturing error. Instead of using an asbestos filter to purify the vaccine, the company used a glass filter because the process was faster. Unknown to the vaccine makers, some bits of cellular material slipped through the glass filter, and clinging to the dead bits of cells were live polio viruses that hid and escaped death by formaldehyde. The contaminated vaccine was injected into more than 100,000 children. Not only did many of the children contract polio, but they infected others who had not yet been vaccinated. In the end, 70,000 people got polio because of the bad vaccine, 200 were paralyzed, and 10 died. It was the one and only incidence of a human-made epidemic in human history, but it led to improved FDA regulations and safety standards for vaccine manufacturing.

testing has been done before human testing will be allowed. University of California at Davis professor Lynette A. Hart has described some of the safety concerns that are addressed in animals during the first testing of vaccines. She explains that first it is essential to determine that the vaccine cannot cause the disease it is supposed to prevent. With either viruses or bacteria, this means ensuring that the pathogens are completely inactivated and that none have survived the killing methods. Researchers must also determine that no pathogens or microorganisms have accidentally been introduced into the vaccine. For example, a vaccine produced by growing the pathogen in animal cells could include an undetected virus hiding in the cells that might cause infection when the vaccine is injected. Any such pathogen could be detected by researchers in their test animals when they check the animals' blood for specific antibodies to the target disease. Antibodies to different diseases would indicate a problem, as would symptoms of an unexpected illness.

Animal testing today involves measuring the number of antibodies produced in response to the vaccine. Researchers can determine with blood tests whether enough antibodies are produced to protect against the specific disease. Then they experiment with giving the test animals unusually high doses of the vaccines in multiple injections. This procedure assures that even large doses do not cause symptoms of illness or serious side effects. It is a way of determining that cancer cells are not triggered by the introduction of foreign material into the body. If at any time animals become ill, the vaccine testing is halted and no human tests are begun.

Animal Testing Controversy

The vast majority of scientists and 97 percent of medical doctors agree with the FDA that animal testing is essential in medical research and for developing new vaccines. Yet modern researchers also recognize that the animals should be ethically and humanely treated. In the United States this means, at minimum, following the guidelines of the 1966 Animal Welfare Act from the U.S. Department of Agriculture concerning basic living conditions, health care, and proper food. Furthermore, both pharmaceutical companies and research laboratories say that they strive to perform their animal testing ethically. At GlaxoSmithKline, for example, company policy requires that the number of animals in experiments be held to the minimum necessary for good science, that animals not be subjected to unnecessary pain or suffering, and that the animals be well cared for throughout their lives. At most university research centers, such as Tufts University in New England, all experiments involving animals are reviewed and must be approved by a university oversight committee or ethics panel. Nevertheless, animals can suffer pain, illness, or death when new drugs or vaccines are tested.

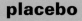

placebo

A substance containing no medication or active treatment that is used during experimental research. It is given to one group of people in the trial, while another group receives the actual treatment.

Harming animals for the benefit of humans is, in the view of some people, both unnecessary and cruel, even when the animals survive. The experimental 2009 H1N1 vaccine, for example, was tested first in mice and ferrets. Ferrets were chosen because they are considered most similar to people in the way their bodies react to influenza viruses. One group of ferrets was given the new vaccine and another was given a placebo, which in this case was a

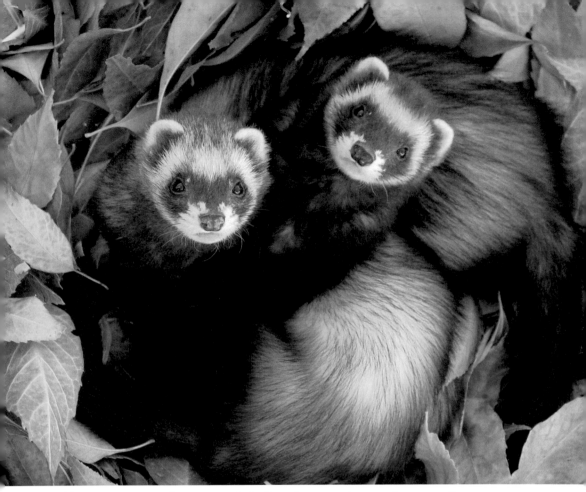

Vaccines are tested on animals before they are given to humans. Because ferrets (pictured) react to influenza viruses similarly to people, one type of H1N1 vaccine was tested first on ferrets.

vaccine look-alike that actually contained no vaccine. Then all the ferrets were exposed to the H1N1 virus. None of the vaccinated ferrets got sick, but those that got the placebo showed the symptoms of flu infection. Although all of the ferrets recovered, half did get sick, and all were subjected to the pain of injections.

Some animal rights organizations argue that such treatment exploits animals and is immoral. People for the Ethical Treatment of Animals (PETA) and In Defense of Animals (IDA), for example, argue that all animal testing should be outlawed. The IDA states on its Web site: "No lab rat (or dog or monkey) ever signed a consent form. In and of itself, this constitutes an ethical problem with the practice of experimenting on non-human animals for the hypothetical benefit of humans."[37] The IDA insists that animal studies cannot predict the efficacy or safety of vaccines in humans. PETA generally echoes these assertions and adds that important medical developments from animal testing could have been achieved by different means.

Americans for Medical Progress, a nonprofit organization supported by medical schools and research institutions, vehemently disagrees. On its Web site it says: "Animal research plays a crucial role in scientists' understanding of diseases and in the development of effective medical treatments. . . . Animals are biologically similar to humans in many ways and they are vulnerable to over 200 of the same health problems. This makes them an effective model for researchers to study."[38] Vaccine researchers also explain that there are no laboratory alternatives today to animal testing of newly developed drugs and vaccines. Because of animal research, argue scientists, thousands of human lives have been saved, and therefore animal testing is justifiable, despite ethical concerns.

Moving to Human Trials

As critical as animal testing is for vaccine development, the time comes when human testing is necessary. In the United States the process is a series of tests called clinical trials. When researchers or pharmaceutical companies want to perform human trials for a new vaccine, they must submit an Investigational New Drug application to the FDA. The application describes the method used to develop the vaccine, preliminary animal test results, and an explanation of the target population (age, gender, and so on) on which the vaccine will be tested. Once approved, clinical trials are done in three phases that may take as long as 10 years to complete. In each phase vaccine researchers monitor and collect data for every person enrolled in the trial. Phase 1 trials involve a small number of people and concentrate on safety and whether an immune response can be identified. Phase 2 trials involve several hundred people and often are used to establish ideal doses of the vaccine, both for safety and for the best antibody response. Phase 3 trials involve thousands of people and include carefully kept scientific records for all trial participants about any side effects, safety issues, and the efficacy of the vaccine. (The meningitis A vaccine currently being tested in India is in Phase 3 trials.)

clinical trials

In medical research, testing of a new drug or vaccine for safety and effectiveness by monitoring the effects on a group of people. Usually these people are volunteers.

Janet Woodcock

Janet Woodcock is the director of the Center for Drug Evaluation and Research in the U.S. Food and Drug Administration (FDA) and is in charge of overseeing the government's approval of any drugs and vaccines. Her center is responsible for approving and evaluating clinical trials, providing use and safety information about drugs to health professionals, regulating drug-making standards, and determining that any drugs (including vaccines) work as they are supposed to and provide health benefits that are greater than the risks of any known side effects.

Woodcock attended Northwestern University Medical School and then taught at Pennsylvania University and the University of California at San Francisco. She joined the FDA in 1986 and became the director of the Center for Drug Evaluation and Research in 1994. In her role as director, Woodcock has been criticized by some people, especially pharmaceutical companies, who complain that she is too conservative where safety is concerned. These critics say she is slow to approve new drugs, citing the fact that she delayed approval of the human papillomavirus vaccine, for instance, when European countries approved it quickly. Woodcock, however, refuses to lower her standards. She takes her job as a guardian of the public health seriously and believes in "safety first." She says, "I am continually challenged to make sure that FDA's regulatory process remains the world's gold standard for drug approval and safety."

Quoted in U.S. Food and Drug Administration, "Meet Janet Woodcock, M.D., Director, Center for Drug Evaluation and Research," January 11, 2010. www.fda.gov.

If concerns about safety arise at any stage, the FDA or the researchers conducting the trials can order that the trials be halted. For example, in 2010 Merck was testing a new vaccine to help the immune system fight lung cancer in a Phase 2 trial with 30 volunteers. Then, one of the volunteers developed encephalitis (an inflammation of the brain). This illness is so serious that on March 23, Merck immediately halted the trial until the researchers could investigate the problem and be absolutely sure that the vaccine did not cause the encephalitis.

Assuming all goes well with clinical trials, however, an application for final approval is submitted to the FDA. Once the vaccine is licensed, the FDA conducts safety inspections of the manufacturing plant for the vaccine and must approve the labeling information so that doctors will know the appropriate doses and any contraindications (circumstances in which the drug may do harm) for use. When the vaccine is finally in public use, the FDA still monitors its safety. Doctors and other medical personnel will submit reports of suspected side effects or safety concerns to the FDA through its Vaccine Adverse Event Reporting System. This system is necessary because, according to the CDC, "until a vaccine is given to the general population, all potential adverse events cannot be anticipated."[39]

contraindications

In medicine, conditions or factors that make a treatment or procedure (such as vaccination) inadvisable because it may be harmful.

A Clinical Trials Failure

Sometimes, despite all the extensive care and testing involved in developing a new vaccine, a dangerous side effect is not found until after a vaccine has been approved. Usually this involves a very rare reaction. A vaccine against the rotavirus, which leads to serious gastrointestinal illness in young children, caused just such a rare complication. Rotavirus is not usually a fatal illness, but it is a major cause of diarrhea, which can result in death by dehydration among people who are not promptly treated. It causes disease by infecting cells in the small intestine. In the United States rotavirus causes only about 100 deaths a year, but around the world, especially in developing countries, it is responsible for about 1 million deaths a year. Most fatalities are in children under five years old.

RotaShield, an attenuated vaccine for rotavirus, was FDA approved in 1998 after extensive and complete clinical trails. However, a year later, in October 1999, Wyeth withdrew its vaccine from the market permanently. The CDC had discovered a serious problem. Once the vaccine was being used in the general population, health professionals reported 76 cases of intussusception. Intussusception is an obstruction of the bowel and can be fatal if not medically or surgically treated. Even though it occurs in no more than one in 5,000 children, it is too dangerous to risk this possible serious side effect when U.S. children rarely die of rotavirus infections anyway.

Continual Monitoring Needed

Since that time, two other rotavirus vaccines have been developed, and the CDC collected data on the incidence of intussusception in babies vaccinated with these new vaccines. It found no greater incidence of intussusception in vaccinated children than in unvaccinated ones. Still, the makers of the new vaccines continued to report every case of intestinal blockage and to conduct safety studies among thousands of children worldwide.

In 2009 experts estimated that these vaccines could prevent at least 228,000 childhood deaths each year in the developing world, and WHO recommended that rotavirus vaccines be included in all national immunization programs. Nevertheless, on March 22, 2010, the FDA recommended that U.S. doctors stop using one of the vaccines, called Rotarix. Researchers discovered that the vaccine was contaminated with a virus that infects pigs. Although the virus has never infected humans, researchers are worried and must determine if the contamination is with whole viruses or just fragments. Theoretically, the virus particles could cause infection and illness.

Vaccines and Public Perceptions

In the United States the CDC lists 27 different diseases for which there are vaccines and recommends 11 of these vaccines for children between birth and 6 years old. This includes 2 vaccines that protect against multiple pathogens: the DTaP vaccine (which protects against diphtheria, tetanus, and pertussis) and the MMR vaccine (which protects against measles, mumps, and rubella). Vaccine researchers have extensively tested all these vaccines according to FDA guidelines. The CDC says, "Vaccines are held to the highest standards of safety." Nevertheless, states the CDC, "there may be rare side effects or delayed reactions that may be detected only after the vaccine is given to millions of people after it is licensed and recommended. However, a decision not to immunize a child also involves risk. It is a decision to put the child and others who come into contact with him or her at risk of getting a disease that could be deadly."[40]

Some preventable diseases are reemerging in the developed world because some people have become more frightened of certain vaccines than of the risk of disease. This is the case especially with the MMR

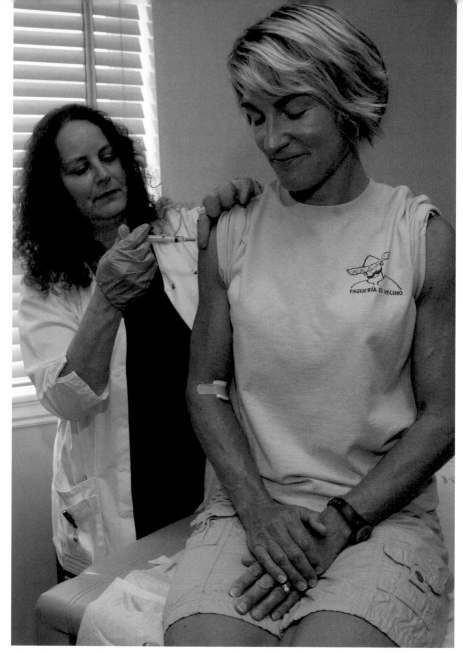

A volunteer takes part in a vaccine clinical trial. In the United States, all new vaccines undergo three phases of clinical trials during which increasingly larger groups of volunteers are immunized and monitored.

vaccine, which, according to the CDC, is feared because of misinformation and unscientific reports about illnesses that coincidentally set in at the same time as a vaccination. Some parents and antivaccine activists believe that the MMR vaccine can cause autism and intestinal disease in young children.

Bad Science, Fear, and Disease Risk

The theory that the MMR vaccine can cause autism began in 1998 in England with physician Andrew Wakefield, who claimed that the MMR vaccine had caused intestinal inflammation in some of his patients that had, in turn, poisoned their brains and caused autism. Wakefield had no evidence of why the MMR vaccine would cause autism; he had only stories of children becoming autistic after vaccination, but one theory blamed a preservative in the vaccine named thimerosal. Although repeated studies provided evidence that thimerosal is safe, it was eliminated from the vaccine in 1999 because of public concerns. The incidence of autism since that time has not increased or decreased, suggesting that autism is unrelated to either thimerosal or vaccination.

In 2010 the British medical journal *The Lancet*, which had published Wakefield's paper about the connection, retracted the study, saying that Wakefield's research had not been honest and was not scientifically accurate. CDC scientists were pleased by *The Lancet*'s statement. The scientists said, "It builds on the overwhelming body of research by the world's leading scientists that concludes there is no link between MMR vaccine and autism. We want to remind parents that vaccines are very safe and effective and they save lives."[41]

Alison Singer, a mother of an autistic child and president of the Autism Science Foundation, believes Wakefield's assertions damaged not only vaccine researchers but also children. She says, "That study did a lot of harm. People became afraid of vaccinations. This is the Wakefield legacy: this unscientifically grounded fear of vaccinations that result in children dying from vaccine-preventable diseases."[42] After Wakefield's paper was publicized, 100,000 parents in England and Ireland refused to vaccinate their children. An outbreak of measles was the result, and three children died. One of these children was a 14-month-old girl named Naomi. Her mother, Marie, said, "I couldn't believe this could happen. We used to hear about measles, but I never thought that it could be this bad. . . . When she first got sick, the nurse said that it was only the measles. Only?"[43]

"Beyond a Shadow of a Doubt"

In the United States the story of Wakefield's theory also was widely publicized and frightened many people. Paul A. Offit says, "And because it's hard to unring the bell, some parents in the United States, England, and the world still refuse to give the MMR vaccine to their children, fearing that it causes autism."[44] Vaccine researchers tried to refute Wakefield's theory with careful scientific studies of the MMR vaccine, but unsupported stories of the dangers of vaccines—whether MMR or influenza or another vaccine—often spread like wildfire through the media or the Internet.

Princeton University vaccine researcher Adel Mahmoud probably best sums up the attitude of vaccine researchers and medical experts:

> Despite all of society's negative pressures, vaccination has proven itself beyond a shadow of a doubt to be the most logical way to control infectious diseases in a community. The success story is undeniable. There is no measles, a little bit of mumps, no rubella, a little bit of hepatitis B in many communities. And the reason is vaccination. Vaccination is an unbelievably smart way of changing the environment of pathogens in human populations. It is as ecologically important as anything that we have discovered in our long history in the fight between us and microbes. But it's not free. It comes with a price, an imperative. And that is that you have to keep using it.[45]

Innovative Vaccines for the Future

In the 1950s researchers improved upon Louis Pasteur's rabies vaccine and developed a new rabies vaccine that was grown in duck embryos. It was safer than the original vaccine, but the vaccination process was painful and prolonged. It required 23 daily injections in arms, legs, and abdomen over a period of about three weeks. Paul A. Offit says, "The procedure was so torturous that many people feared the vaccine more than they feared rabies."[46] During the 1970s Hilary Koprowski and Tad Wiktor of the Wistar Institute at the University of Pennsylvania improved this rabies vaccine, using human fetal cells. It was safe, 100 percent effective, and required only five injections in the arm.

A Future DNA Vaccine

This same vaccine is still used today, but modern researchers are not satisfied. Rabies still kills about 55,000 people each year around the world, especially in the poorest countries. The vaccine's protection lasts only about 2 years, so people are not immune for life. It must be refrigerated and is expensive. The director of vaccine research at the Wistar Institute, Hildegund C.J. Ertl, and her team have spent 12 years trying to develop an inexpensive, 1-dose rabies vaccine that triggers ample antibody production and provides long-term protection. Their goal is a vaccine that can be given once during childhood and will protect for years.

Ertl's team is working on a DNA vaccine instead of an antigen-based vaccine. It is made with a piece of DNA from a rabies virus that is combined with an adenovirus, a virus that causes respiratory infections in people and animals. The team chose an adenovirus for its genetic engineering because adenoviruses trigger strong immune system responses after just one exposure. They chose to use a piece of DNA from the rabies virus because it codes for only one protein in the virus instead of its complete

DNA, which could be dangerous. The vaccine is called a carrier vaccine, because the harmless virus is *carrying* a piece of the DNA from the pathogen. In tests with nonhuman primates, they found that the vaccine triggers antibodies that last six months. Ertl and her team still have a lot of work to do and are still monitoring their primates, but if they eventually succeed, they will have a cheaply made vaccine that protects people from future rabies bites, while being completely safe.

carrier vaccine

A vaccine preparation using genetic engineering to introduce a gene from a pathogen into a non-disease-causing virus and using that virus to carry the gene into human cells.

So far, however, DNA vaccines have not proved effective in people because they do not always trigger antibodies reliably. The first approved DNA vaccine protects horses from West Nile virus, but human clinical trials are ongoing with DNA vaccines for diseases such as influenza, hepatitis, and prostate cancer. Researchers such as Ertl believe that knowledge about genetic engineering will soon lead them to new DNA vaccines that are cheap, safe, and able to stimulate immunological memory.

The Vaccine Patch

Researchers are continually working to improve old vaccines and to develop new ones. One of the major areas of research involves new delivery systems. Most vaccines are liquids that are injected into tissues with needles and syringes and must be kept refrigerated. This standard injection delivery system is a serious problem in poor countries, where refrigerators, the electrical power to run them, and refrigerated trucks to deliver the vaccines may not be available. Myron Levine, a vaccine expert at the University of Maryland School of Medicine, says, "There is a broad recognition of the need to find ways to administer vaccines without the use of 'sharps' (that is, needles and syringes)."[47]

transcutaneous

Through the unbroken skin.

One of the most promising alternatives to injections is the "vaccine patch." It is a transcutaneous delivery system, meaning "across the skin." Researchers believe that this system would be safe and inexpensive. The patches would not require refrigeration and could be stored in quantity

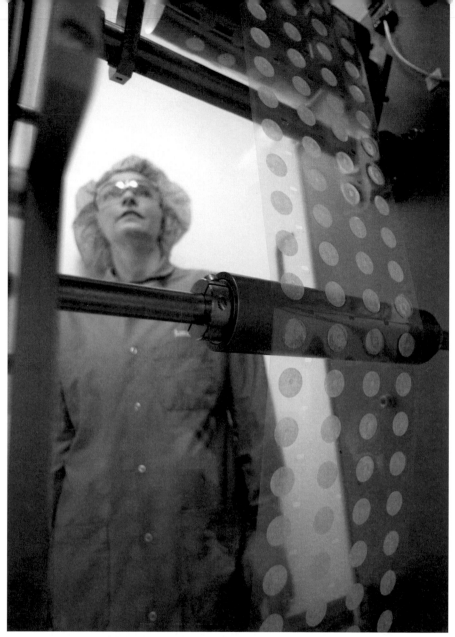

Vaccine patches for influenza roll off a production line under the watchful eye of a plant employee. Vaccine patches, which are still in the testing stage, would not require refrigeration and could be stored in large quantities for future needs.

for future need. Medical personnel would not be needed because people could apply their own patches.

Developing a vaccine patch is difficult because usually the molecules of the vaccine are too large to be absorbed through the skin. In Austria researchers at the company Intercell solve this problem by preparing the

⚛ A Therapeutic Cancer Vaccine

Vaccines today prevent disease but researchers are also trying to develop vaccines that can boost immune system protection for people who are already ill. Such vaccines are called therapeutic vaccines, and in the future they may help in the fight against many cancers. The first such vaccine, called Provenge, was approved by the Food and Drug Administration in 2010 as a treatment for advanced prostate cancer. Scientists explain that every cell in the body has its own "fingerprint," or unique proteins that can be identified. Provenge triggers the immune systems of prostate cancer patients to fight a tumor's fingerprints. About 40 percent of tumor cells produce a protein unique to cancer. It is this protein that the vaccine targets. The vaccine combines a fragment of the tumor protein with chemicals that are known to activate the immune system. White blood cells removed from the patient's blood are mixed with the vaccine in the laboratory. Then these same, cancer-educated blood cells are infused back into the patient where they trigger an immune system attack against the tumor proteins.

Provenge is not a cure but it extends the lives of advanced prostate cancer patients by a median of 4.1 months. The only previous treatment available for late-stage, severely ill prostate cancer patients was a difficult course of chemotherapy that extended lives by only 3 months. And of 512 severely ill patients in a Phase 3 clinical trial of Provenge, 31.7 percent of those treated were still alive after 3 years.

skin before applying the patch. A mildly abrasive substance is first drawn across the skin, making a miniscule dent. One-thousandth of an inch (0.025mm) of skin is removed. Then an adhesive patch containing the vaccine is applied to the spot for a few hours. Intercell has developed a vaccine patch for the type of *Escherichia coli* bacteria that cause traveler's diarrhea. It works by delivering antigens under the skin, where innate immune system cells recognize them as foreign, carry them to the lymph system, and present the antigens to B cells. This sets the immune system response in motion and results in the proliferation of antibodies.

In Phase 2 clinical trials, the patch reduced the risk of traveler's diarrhea by 75 percent. In 2009 Intercell began Phase 3 trials. Herbert

DuPont of the University of Texas is one of the testers of the patch. He says, "I think it's one of the most exciting new developments in travel medicine. . . . People could buy this and put it on themselves whenever they take a trip. It is the most convenient form of immunization I have ever seen."[48]

Dried Vaccines

Convenience and easy storage are also the goals of scientists at Oxford University's Jenner Institute in Great Britain. There Matt Cottingham and his research team are focusing not on needle-free delivery but on dried vaccines. A dried vaccine would not need to be refrigerated and could be transported anywhere. Cottingham says, "If you could ship vaccines at normal temperatures, you would greatly reduce cost and hugely improve access to vaccines. You could even picture someone with a backpack taking vaccine doses on a bike into remote villages."[49]

The team has made great progress in developing such a vaccine. Basically, they mix the vaccine with sugars and leave it to dry on a thin membrane. The mixture turns into a kind of syrup and keeps the vaccine in a kind of "suspended animation." When the membrane is flushed with water, it rehydrates, and the vaccine is ready for injection. Cottingham's team is testing the stability of a vaccine for two different viruses. In 2010 they reported that they could leave the membrane sitting in temperatures of 113°F (45°C) for four to six months without damaging the vaccine. The technology is exciting to fellow researcher Adrian Hill. He explains, "If most or all of the vaccines could be stabilized at high temperatures, it would not only remove cost, more children would be vaccinated."[50]

Toward an AIDS Vaccine

New delivery systems and vaccines that do not need refrigeration could revolutionize global health, but they are only one challenge facing vaccine researchers. Just as important is conquering diseases for which no vaccines are available. An AIDS vaccine has been the goal of researchers for decades. In 2009 the United Nations reported that approximately 33.4 million people worldwide are infected with HIV/AIDS. It is estimated that at least 25 million people have died because of AIDS since 1981. So far, every effort to develop an AIDS vaccine has failed. Some scientists wonder if such a vaccine is even possible, but most have not given up hope for the future.

AIDS (acquired immune deficiency syndrome) is caused by the human immunodeficiency virus (HIV). HIV is a retrovirus consisting of two molecules of RNA, and like all viruses, it hijacks the infected cell's coding in order to replicate. However, HIV specifically infects immune system cells, such as helper T cells and macrophages. The virus kills immune system cells, and when enough immune system cells are destroyed, the person develops an immune deficiency, or full-blown AIDS. At that point, it is easy for other pathogens to invade the body. People with AIDS most often die from opportunistic infections—infections that are able to take hold because the immune system is so weakened by the HIV attack. When HIV first invades, the immune system does recognize the invader and mount an attack; T cells are activated and antibodies form. The immune system, however, is unable to kill all of the viruses. As more and more immune system cells become infected, the immune system finally fails.

retrovirus

Any of the group of viruses with two single-strand RNA molecules that can transfer their genetic coding into the DNA of a cell.

opportunistic infections

Infections that occur because of a weakened immune system.

Developing a vaccine to make the immune system protect itself is difficult. One of the major issues is the question of which kind of memory cells are needed. With most deadly diseases, a few people are able to mount a strong immune response and recover from their infections. For these diseases, scientists can examine the survivor's blood to see whether it was antibodies from B cells or killer T cells or both that won the battle. They can test the "victors," explains Lauren Sompayrac, "to find out which microbial proteins were the targets of the protective immune response."[51] Then they know which kind of vaccine to design or which proteins are the important antigens to include in the vaccine. For HIV this approach is not possible because no one's immune system has ever successfully eliminated the virus. However, most researchers believe that an AIDS vaccine must stimulate production of killer T cells. Only killer T cells can detect and destroy viruses inside cells. Killer T cell production is triggered only by attenuated vaccines, since viruses must be alive to enter cells.

An attenuated HIV vaccine, however, would be much too dangerous. No one would inject a healthy person with live HIV, no matter how weakened the virus was. The chance that one weak but living virus could mutate into an infectious form is too great, and mutation is something that HIV does extremely well. Sompayrac explains, "On average, each AIDS virus produced by an infected cell differs from the original infecting virus by at least one mutation." This very high mutation rate means that HIV develops into many different strains. "Consequently," Sompayrac explains, "the body of someone infected with [HIV] contains not just 'the' AIDS virus but a huge collection of slightly different mutant viruses."[52] Sompayrac believes that this rapid mutation rate is the biggest problem for AIDS vaccine researchers.

Is a DNA Type Vaccine the Answer?

Genetic engineering with an adenovirus, such as Ertl's team is doing with their rabies vaccine, might be a safe way to make an AIDS vaccine. Because the whole, harmless virus with a piece of RNA from HIV is carried into the cell, it could trigger killer T cells without the risk of HIV

A technician in Thailand works with blood samples from volunteers taking part in a clinical trial for an AIDS vaccine. So far the trial, involving more than 16,000 volunteers, has had limited success.

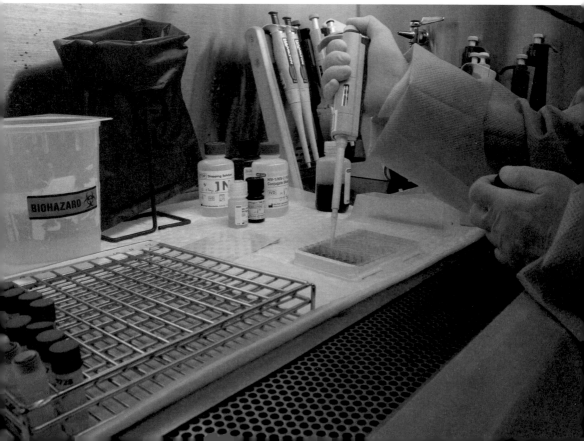

☢ Genes and T Cells

Shane Crotty of the La Jolla Institute in California is a researcher and microbiologist who studies the immune system. He says that scientists still do not understand the immune system well enough to develop completely effective vaccines, and he is trying to change that. In 2009 Crotty led a team that joined with another research team at Yale University to investigate how T cells are activated. The researchers discovered a human gene dubbed BCL6 that acts as an on switch for special helper T cells. It tells white blood cells to become these helper T cells, which in turn activate B cells to produce antibodies. The scientists found another gene, called Blimp 1, that codes for turning off antibody production.

Crotty says that they have uncovered the road map for immune system functioning. Someday, instead of making vaccines from pathogens, researchers might simply make vaccines with chemicals that turn on the BCL6 gene. They might fight autoimmune diseases, in which the immune system mistakenly produces antibodies to its own tissues, with chemicals that activate the Blimp 1 gene. Such vaccines remain far in the future, says Crotty, but, he explains, "We absolutely think that this is a key in the process."

Quoted in Keith Darcé, "Local Researchers Find Key to Vaccines," SignOn San Diego, July 17, 2009. www.signonsandiego.com.

infection. In 2009 researchers at Merck completed Phase 3 clinical trials of just such a vaccine in Thailand. The vaccine targeted two HIV strains common in Thailand. More than 16,000 volunteers took part, receiving either the vaccine or a placebo. Animal studies had already shown that the vaccine reduced the incidence of infection in nonhuman primates when they were vaccinated and then exposed to HIV.

Researchers hoped the vaccine would provide some protection for people, too, but the results were not completely encouraging. Between 2003 and 2009, 74 people who received the placebo became infected with HIV. Of those given the vaccine, 51 were infected. The difference is slight and could be the result of chance instead of any protective effect. So few of the 16,000 people actually were infected by HIV that the trial provides little evidence that the vaccine worked. Nevertheless, Jerome Kim, one of the vaccine researchers, said, "This contributes more evidence that an AIDS vaccine may be possible. We've taken a very small step. It's not a home run, but it opens the door to future work."[53]

Now researchers are examining the volunteers in detail. They are looking for antibodies and T cells in their blood and giving some of the volunteers booster shots to see if the extra doses can increase immunity. They are doing more animal studies to learn if multiple doses work better than single injections. The researchers hope that they will gain enough information to reformulate an AIDS vaccine in the future. Even a vaccine that protects against just a few HIV strains could save many lives.

Malaria Vaccines

AIDS is not the only disease for which a vaccine has proved elusive. No one has ever developed a vaccine against a parasite, but a future malaria vaccine might be the first. Worldwide, malaria kills about 1 million people a year. Although adults build up some natural immunity over years of repeated exposure to the parasite, children often die from the disease. Malaria is caused by the bites of mosquitoes infected by the microscopic malaria parasite. The parasite is injected into a person when he or she is bitten; it then travels to the liver, multiplies, and develops into a new form. The new forms then infect red blood cells. The parasites multiply inside red blood cells, burst out, and go on to infect more blood cells. When a malaria victim is bitten by another mosquito, the blood forms of the parasites are taken in with the mosquito's blood meal. Now the life cycle is completed inside the infected mosquito, as thousands of parasitic eggs or spores hatch and grow in the mosquito until they can infect the next person the mosquito bites.

The complex life cycle of the malaria parasite makes vaccine development a challenge, but researchers believe they are close to success. The Malaria Vaccine Initiative, of the Program for Appropriate Technology in Health, has set the goal of designing the first malaria vaccine by 2015. An effective vaccine has to interrupt the parasite's life cycle, but scientists still do not understand how the immune system protects against parasites; at each stage in the life cycle, there are thousands of protein antigens for the immune system to recognize. Which antigens should be in a vaccine is not yet known. Currently, some vaccine efforts focus on the liver stage of the parasite, some on the blood stage, and some on the mosquito itself.

Promising Possibilities

In 2010 GlaxoSmithKline researcher Christopher Plowe and his team tested a blood stage vaccine with 100 children in Mali. The vaccine is made of protein antigens from the surface of the blood form of the parasite combined with an adjuvant. An adjuvant is a chemical compound that helps boost immune system response. With malaria the adjuvant is necessary because the immune system makes antibodies naturally to the antigens of the blood form of the parasite only after repeated exposures and infections. The vaccine did not prevent initial infection, but the blood form of the disease is what sickens and kills, and Plowe reported that the children's antibodies against the blood form increased "100-fold." Plowe said, "The antibody levels that the vaccinated children achieved were as high or higher than those measured in adults whose lifelong exposure to malaria protects them against the disease."[54] Plowe's team is now testing the vaccine in a larger group of Malian children.

adjuvant

Any chemical added to a drug or vaccine to increase its effect.

The Malaria Vaccine Initiative is working on a different, transmission-blocking vaccine. It is a vaccine given to people but targeting the transmission of the parasite from mosquitoes to people. The idea is that when a mosquito bites a vaccinated person, the mosquito takes up the vaccine proteins in its blood meal. The proteins are antibodies to the molecules in a mosquito's gut that the parasites have to invade in order to grow. Inside the mosquito, the vaccine prevents any malaria parasite from finding those molecules and growing, and that makes a mosquito bite harmless to people.

The most promising proposed malaria vaccine, from researchers at GlaxoSmithKline, targets the liver form of malaria. It is genetically engineered with proteins from the malaria parasite's liver stage of development and an antigen from the hepatitis B virus's surface. It triggers macrophages to attack and causes a full immune system response, including memory B cells and T cells. During Phase 2 trials, the vaccine was found to be about 50 percent effective in preventing malaria symptoms. Phase 3 trials of this vaccine in seven African countries will continue into 2011. No one knows which approach is best for an effective malaria vaccine. No malaria vaccine has moved beyond trials yet, but, explains one researcher, Filip Dubovsky, "We're absolutely certain that a malaria vaccine is feasible."[55]

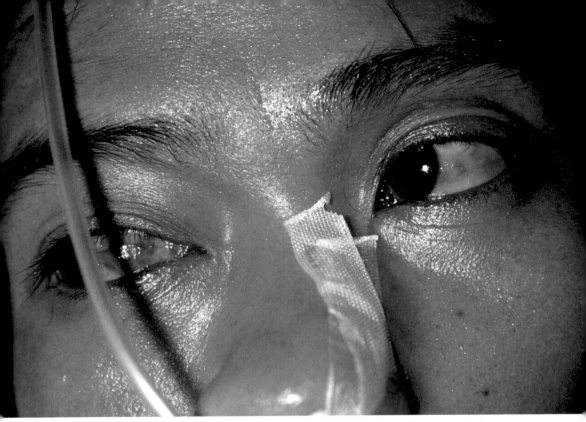

A patient in Vietnam shows signs of malaria including yellowing of the skin and the whites of the eyes. Researchers have been trying to develop a vaccine against malaria, an often-deadly illness caused by a mosquito-borne parasite.

The Need for a Tuberculosis Vaccine

Vaccine researchers are also confident that they can develop a vaccine against another major worldwide killer—tuberculosis (TB). TB kills about 1.8 million people every year, and approximately one-third of the world's people are infected with the bacterium. Although medical treatment can cure TB, it is a months-long, expensive process, not available to many of the world's poor. Scientists believe that a TB vaccine is urgently needed.

Although TB can infect any body organ, *Mycobacterium tuberculosis* most often invades macrophages in the lungs after it is breathed in from an infected person. When it first settles in the lungs, it is immediately recognized as a foreign invader and attacked, but when a macrophage engulfs the bacterium, the pathogen does not die. The hard capsule surrounding the bacterium protects it from the macrophage's pouch of killing chemicals. Inside the macrophage, the TB bacterium feeds and multiplies. When the bacteria burst from the macrophage, killing it, the destructive chemicals are spilled into the lungs, where they damage tissues instead of invaders. This process continues as the immune system battles the multiplying bacteria, and the bacteria invade more and more macrophages. Although the immune system cannot destroy the bacteria, it does sometimes fight to a tie that may last for decades. It keeps the bacteria walled off and unable to replicate. The person has latent TB and no symptoms. When the immune system loses, however, damage is so severe that the person will die without medical treatment.

Slow Progress

So far, efforts to provide sustained immunity with a TB vaccine have failed. An old TB vaccine, called BCG, is made from a TB bacterial strain that infects cattle and is similar to the bacterium that causes human TB. It provides partial protection in infants, but it cannot protect against lung infections, does nothing for latent TB, and is unsafe for people with HIV infection. TB, as an opportunistic infection, kills more people with AIDS than any other disease. The efforts to develop an effective TB vaccine are not as advanced as for a malaria vaccine, but the nonprofit Aeras Global TB Vaccine Foundation does report progress. It is supporting research into six different kinds of TB vaccines.

Research suggests that a technique called "prime-boosting" may be the best strategy against TB. Prime-boosting is a strategy of priming the immune system so that the antigens from a first dose of one vaccine (perhaps given in infancy) are boosted with doses of another vaccine at a later time (in adulthood). For example, Aeras researchers conducted a trial with African adults who were given the BCG vaccine in infancy. They were no longer protected against TB. The researchers boosted the BCG vaccination by administering a new vaccine called Aeras-402, which combines antigens from the bacterium with a weakened adenovirus. In 2010 the research team reported that tests showed immune system activation and the triggering of T cells in the vaccinated people.

In another trial of prime-boosting, Dartmouth Medical School scientists developed a vaccine with a different strain of mycobacterium called *Mycobacterium vaccae*. It has antigens in common with *Mycobacterium tuberculosis* and is killed with heat. They gave this vaccine to half of a group of 2,000 African people already infected with HIV who had also received BCG in infancy. In 2010, after three years, the researchers reported a 39 percent decrease of TB infections in the people who received the vaccine as compared to those who were given a placebo. The vaccine did not provide 100 percent protection, but, said researcher Richard Waddell, "This is the first TB vaccine to show effectiveness in any clinical trial. It will re-energize the search for an even more effective TB vaccine, which is especially urgent in Africa."[56]

"Decade of Vaccines"

The Bill and Melinda Gates Foundation says that new vaccines for the developing world are one of 14 grand challenges for humanity's future. TB, malaria, and AIDS alone take 5 million lives every year. Urges Bill Gates, "We must make this the decade of vaccines. Vaccines already save and improve millions of lives in developing countries. Innovation will make it possible to save more children than ever before."[57] To that end, the Gates Foundation and other nonprofit organizations support vaccine researchers in their quest for effective, affordable vaccines, not just for developed countries, but to change the futures of all people everywhere.

Source Notes

Introduction: To Save Lives

1. Centers for Disease Control and Prevention, "How Vaccines Prevent Disease." www.cdc.gov.

2. Michael Good, "Promises and Challenges in Developing New Vaccines, with a Focus on Diseases of the Developing World," *ANU News*, Australian National University, April 29, 2009. www.anu.edu.au.

Chapter One: What Are Vaccines?

3. National Institute of Allergy and Infectious Diseases, "Understanding the Immune System: How It Works," U.S. Department of Health and Human Services, National Institutes of Health, NIH Publication No. 07-5423, September 2007, p. 27.

4. Lauren Sompayrac, *How the Immune System Works*. 3rd ed. Malden, MA: Blackwell, 2008, p. 3.

5. Sompayrac, *How the Immune System Works*, pp. 6–7.

6. Sompayrac, *How the Immune System Works*, p. 11.

7. Sompayrac, *How the Immune System Works*, p. 96.

8. Quoted in Paul A. Offit, *Vaccinated: One Man's Quest to Defeat the World's Deadliest Diseases*. NY: HarperCollins, 2008, p. 30.

Chapter Two: Vaccines and Viruses

9. Quoted in Offit, *Vaccinated*, p. 67.

10. Quoted in Offit, *Vaccinated*, p. 67.

11. Corey Binns, "Inside Look: How Viruses Invade Us," Live Science, June 5, 2006. www.livescience.com.

12. Binns, "Inside Look."

13. Quoted in Lawrence C. Paoletti and Pamela M. McInnes, eds., *Vaccines from Concept to Clinic: A Guide to the Development and Clinical Testing of Vaccines for Human Use*. Boca Raton, FL: CRC, 1999, p. 184.

14. Quoted in Offit, *Vaccinated*, p. 102.

15. Vaccine Education Center, "How Are Vaccines Made?" Children's Hospital of Philadelphia, March 2008. www.chop.edu.

16. Debi Vinnedge, "Responding to the Call: Is Anyone Listening?" LifeIssues.net, August 10, 2005. www.lifeissues.net.

17. National Network for Immunization Information, "Vaccine Components: Human Fetal Links with Some Vaccines," June 3, 2008. www.immunizationinfo.org.

18. Jacqueline Jaeger Houtman, "Viruses, Cancer, Warts, and All: The HPV Vaccine for Cervical Cancer," *Breakthroughs in Bioscience*, Federation of American Societies for Experimental Biology, p. 14. www.faseb.org.

19. Houtman, "Viruses, Cancer, Warts, and All," p. 14.

20. Quoted in Corydon Ireland, "A Cancer Vaccine Is Born," *Rochester Review*, University of Rochester, Spring 2006. www.rochester.edu.

21. Offit, *Vaccinated*, p. 3.

22. Quoted in Daniel J. DeNoon, "Swine Flu Vaccine: The Race Is On," MedicineNet.com, June 26, 2009. www.medicinenet.com.

23. Quoted in Todd Zwillich, "Swine Flu Vaccine by October, Say Makers," Rx List, July 23, 2009. www.rxlist.com.

24. Quoted in Tom Corwin, "VLP Could Make Flu Vaccine Faster, Better," *Augusta Chronicle*, September 20, 2009. http://chronicle.augusta.com.

25. Quoted in Corwin, "VLP Could Make Flu Vaccine Faster, Better."

26. Quoted in Maggie Fox, "WHO Expects H1N1 Virus to Lurk," *Emirates Business*, February 25, 2010. www.business24-7.ae.

Chapter Three: Vaccines and Bacteria

27. Toni McCaffery and David McCaffery, "An Open Letter from Toni and David McCaffery," Dana McCaffery.com. http://danamccaffery.com.

28. Offit, *Vaccinated*, p. 143.

29. Quoted in Offit, *Vaccinated*, p. 154.

30. Quoted in Ronald J. Eby, Dace V. Madore, and Velupillai Puvane-sarajah, "The Story of Prevnar," Innovation.org. www.innovation.org.

31. Quoted in World Pharma News, "Pfizer's Prevnar 13 Recommended by CDC's Advisory Committee on Immunization Practices," February 25, 2010. www.worldpharmanews.com.

32. Quoted in Melissa Dahl, "Killer at College: Meningitis Threatens Students," MSNBC, September 5, 2007. MSNBC. www.msnbc.msn.com.

33. Quoted in Meningitis Vaccine Project, "Why Is There No Vaccine Suitable for Africa?" 2010. www.meningvax.org.

34. Meningitis Vaccine Project, "Vaccine Introduction," 2010. www.meningvax.org.

35. Meningitis Vaccine Project, "Measuring Success," 2010. www.meningvax.org.

Chapter Four: Safe, Effective, and Approved

36. Quoted in Offit, *Vaccinated*, p. 35.

37. The Truth About Vivisection, "Frequently Asked Questions." www.vivisectioninfo.org.

38. Americans for Medical Progress, "Animal Research," 2010. www.amprogress.org.

39. Centers for Disease Control and Prevention, "Vaccine Product Approval Process," August 2001. www.hhs.gov.

40. Centers for Disease Control and Prevention, "Vaccine Safety," April 20, 2009. www.cdc.gov.

41. Quoted in Madison Park, "Medical Journal Retracts Study Linking Autism to Vaccine," CNN, February 2, 2010. www.cnn.com.

42. Quoted in Park, "Medical Journal Retracts Study Linking Autism to Vaccine."

43. Quoted in Offit, *Vaccinated*, p. 163.

44. Offit, *Vaccinated*, p. 170.

45. Quoted in Offit, *Vaccinated*, pp. 184–85.

Chapter Five: Innovative Vaccines for the Future

46. Offit, *Vaccinated*, p. 101.

47. Quoted in Health WorldNet, "Needle and Pain Free Vaccinations," April 5, 2009. http://healthworldnet.com.

48. Quoted in Health WorldNet, "Needle and Pain Free Vaccinations."

49. Quoted in Kate Kelland, "Sugar Technology Keeps Vaccines Stable in the Heat," Reuters Africa, February 18, 2010. http://af.reuters.com.

50. Quoted in Kelland, "Sugar Technology Keeps Vaccines Stable in the Heat."

51. Sompayrac, *How the Immune System Works*, p. 97.

52. Sompayrac, *How the Immune System Works*, p. 99.

53. Quoted in Katherine Harmon, "Renewed Hope for an AIDS Vaccine," *Scientific American*, November 16, 2009. www.scientificamerican.com.

54. Quoted in Howard Hughes Medical Institute, "New Vaccine Shows Promise Against Malaria in Early-Stage Study," February 4, 2010. www.hhmi.org.

55. Quoted in Tom Paulson, "Gates Foundation Fighting Malaria a World Away," *Seattle Post-Intelligencer*, July 17, 2003. www.seattlepi.com.

56. Quoted in PlusNews, "Africa: High Hopes as New TB Vaccine Proves Effective," February 11, 2010. www.plusnews.org.

57. Quoted in Bill & Melinda Gates Foundation, "Bill and Melinda Gates Pledge $10 Billion in Call for Decade of Vaccines," January 29, 2010. www.gatesfoundation.org.

Facts About Vaccines

Immune System

- Close to 99 percent of all animals have just an innate immune system. Vertebrates are the only animals (including humans) that have developed an adaptive immune system to protect them against invaders.
- In a healthy person there are about 7,000 to 25,000 white blood cells in a drop of blood. This number increases dramatically when the immune system is fighting disease.
- White blood cells live between five and nine days.
- Immune system expert Philip Tierno Jr. says that getting enough sleep strengthens the immune system, but no one knows exactly how.
- The human body has about 500 to 700 lymph nodes. Most are about 0.4 inches (1cm) in size, but when the immune system is activated, a lymph node swells 2 to 4 times bigger because white blood cells are multiplying.

Infectious Diseases

- The influenza epidemic of 1918 to 1919 was the last great plague, infecting one-half (500 million people) of the world's population and killing between 50 and 100 million.
- As of 2010 scientists estimate that about 20 percent of all cancers are the result of cancer-causing gene mutations caused by viral infections and, therefore, may be preventable with future vaccines.
- According to the Global Health Council, infectious diseases cause more than 9.5 million deaths each year, almost all in developing countries.
- According to the World Health Organization, 50 percent of all premature deaths are caused by just six infectious diseases—pneumonia, tuberculosis, diarrheal diseases, malaria, measles, and AIDS.

Pathogens

- The bacteria that cause tuberculosis are released into the air when an infected person coughs, talks, or sneezes, and they can remain suspended in the air for several hours, ready to infect anyone who inhales them.

- The virus that causes hepatitis A can survive outside the human body for months, but HIV is a fragile virus that cannot survive outside the body, exposed to the air, for more than a few hours.
- Measles is the most contagious disease known to humanity, but according to the Red Cross, it can be prevented by a vaccination that costs less than $1.
- Cold and flu viruses in the water droplets of a sneeze can travel up to 3 feet (0.9m).
- Of the 2,000 known species of bacteria in the world, 99 percent are either harmless or beneficial, and less than 1 percent cause disease.
- In 2010 researchers in Australia at the University of New South Wales discovered two new, mutated strains of pertussis bacteria, and the scientists are concerned that today's whooping cough vaccine may not be effective against them.

Immunization

- According to the Board on Health Care Services of the Institute of Medicine, vaccines account for just 1.5 percent of worldwide pharmaceutical sales.
- A Centers for Disease Control and Prevention survey of U.S. teens between 13 and 17 years old determined that in 2008, 18 percent of girls had received all 3 recommended doses of the human papillomavirus (HPV) vaccine.
- According to the Centers for Disease Control and Prevention, global incidence of polio has decreased from 350,000 cases in 1988, when global eradication efforts began with vaccination, to 2,000 cases in 2006. Polio has been successfully eliminated in Europe, the Western Hemisphere, and the Western Pacific.
- The Centers for Disease Control and Prevention reports that in 1921, 15,520 U.S. deaths occurred from diphtheria. In 2001 only two cases were reported, neither of them fatal.
- Because of successful vaccination programs, smallpox was eliminated from the United States in 1972 and worldwide by 1980. The "wild" virus is eradicated, but, according to the Centers for Disease Control and Prevention, stocks of the virus continue to live in research laboratories in the United States and Russia.
- In 2006 economists Christopher P. Adams and Van V. Brantner estimated that the cost to bring a new drug or vaccine to the market ranges from $500 million to $2 billion.

- In 2008, according to the World Health Organization, 108 million children worldwide received all routine immunizations, but 24 million children did not receive any recommended vaccinations.
- Since 1983 the Centers for Disease Control and Prevention has maintained stockpiles of essential vaccines to protect U.S. children in case of infectious disease outbreaks or vaccine shortages. The stockpiles include supplies of MMR (measles, mumps, rubella), chickenpox, polio, tetanus, and other vaccines equal to the amount needed to vaccinate every child in the United States during a six-month period.

Related Organizations

Aeras Global TB Vaccine Foundation

1405 Research Blvd.
Rockville, MD 20850
phone: (301) 547-2900
Web site: www.aeras.org

Aeras is a nonprofit organization with the mission of developing, licensing, manufacturing, and distributing at least one tuberculosis vaccine for infants and another for teens that will be affordable and available worldwide.

Bill & Melinda Gates Foundation

PO Box 23350
Seattle, WA 98102
phone: (206) 709-3100
Web site: www.gatesfoundation.org

The Gates Foundation is a philanthropic organization that has provided major funding for vaccine research and distribution in the developing world. The foundation has pledged $10 billion for new vaccine development, calling it a critical global need for the twenty-first century.

Centers for Disease Control and Prevention (CDC)

1600 Clifton Rd.
Atlanta, GA 30333
phone: (800) 232-4636
Web site: www.cdc.gov

The CDC provides extensive, up-to-date information about vaccines, vaccination, and infectious diseases.

Doctors Without Borders (MSF USA)

333 Seventh Ave., 2nd Floor
New York, NY 10001-5004

phone: (212) 679-6800
Web site: www.doctorswithoutborders.org

Dedicated to providing emergency medical assistance in 70 countries throughout the world, Médecins Sans Frontières (or Doctors Without Borders) is a leading advocate of bringing effective, affordable vaccines to developing countries.

Institute for Vaccine Safety

Johns Hopkins Bloomberg School of Public Health
615 N. Wolfe St., Room W5041
Baltimore, MD 21205
Web site: www.vaccinesafety.edu

Established by the Johns Hopkins University School of Public Health, this educational organization's goal is to prevent disease with the safest possible vaccines.

National Foundation for Infectious Diseases (NFID)

4733 Bethesda Ave., Suite 750
Bethesda, MD 20814
phone: (301) 656-0003
Web site: www.nfid.org

The NFID is a nonprofit organization dedicated to educating the public and health-care professionals about the cause, treatment, and prevention of infectious disease.

National Network for Immunization Information (NNii)

301 University Blvd.
Galveston, TX 77555-0350
phone: (409) 772-0199
Web site: www.immunizationinfo.org

The NNii is an affiliation of several medical and health-care organizations dedicated to providing scientifically accurate information and education about immunizations.

Program for Appropriate Technology in Health (PATH)

PO Box 900922
Seattle, WA 98109

phone: (206) 285-3500
Web site: www.path.org

PATH is a global nonprofit organization and cofounder of the Meningitis Vaccine Project in Africa and of the Malaria Vaccine Initiative.

U.S. Food and Drug Administration (FDA)
10903 New Hampshire Ave.
Silver Spring, MD 20993-0002
phone: (888) 463-6332
Web site: www.fda.gov

The FDA is the federal government's regulatory agency for evaluating and approving vaccine research, vaccine safety, and new vaccines. Consult the Web site section "Vaccines, Blood & Biologics" for more information.

Vaccination Liberation
PO Box 457
Spirit Lake, ID 83869-0457
phone: (888) 249-1421
Web site: www.vaclib.org

This group describes itself as a grassroots organization fighting the myth that vaccines are safe, effective, or necessary to prevent disease.

For Further Research

Books

Sylvia Engdahl, *Vaccines.* Detroit, MI: Greenhaven, 2008.

Louise I. Gerdes, *The Pharmaceutical Industry.* Detroit, MI: Greenhaven, 2008.

Connie Goldsmith, *Meningitis.* Minneapolis, MN: Twenty-First Century, 2008.

Victoria Sherrow, *Jonas Salk: Beyond the Microscope.* 2nd rev. ed. New York: Chelsea House, 2008.

Gregory J. Stewart, *The Immune System.* New York: Chelsea House, 2009.

Web Sites

The Big Picture Book of Viruses (www.virology.net/Big_Virology/ BVHomePage.html). From virologists at Tulane University, this site is a catalog of actual electron microscope photographs and descriptions of viruses, organized by virus families, infectious disease, hosts, and individual name.

Immunisation (www.immunisation.nhs.uk). This Web site from the United Kingdom's National Health Service uses animations, pictures, and text to describe how vaccines are made, why they are important, and which vaccines are recommended in the United Kingdom. It also provides up-to-date information about the latest immunization news.

International AIDS Vaccine Initiative (www.iavi.org/Pages/home. aspx). Visitors to this Web site can learn about the urgent need for an AIDS vaccine and the ongoing research efforts to develop a vaccine. Click the links to learn about new antibody discoveries and ongoing clinical trials.

On Being a Scientist: A Guide to Responsible Conduct in Research (www.nap.edu/openbook.php?record_id=12192&page=R1). This is a free, downloadable book from the National Academy of Sciences Committee on Science, Engineering, and Public Policy. The 2009 edition provides a clear explanation of the responsible conduct of scientific research. Chapters on treatment of data, mistakes and negligence, the scientist's role in society, and other topics offer invaluable insight for student researchers.

Virtual Museum of Bacteria (www.bacteriamuseum.org). From the Foundation of Bacteriology and the Society of Applied Microbiology, this large site explores bacteria—whether benign or harmful—in depth. Follow the links for Pathogenic Bacteria to learn about diseases, vaccines, and the immune system. Many images of different kinds of bacteria are available, too.

Wistar Institute (www.wistar.org). Founded in 1892, this nonprofit research institute is dedicated to medical research and the discovery of new processes for the treatment and prevention of disease. At the Vaccine Center, visitors can explore past vaccine successes and current research efforts, as well as learn about the scientists at the institute.

Index

Picture Credits

Cover: iStockphoto.com
Maury Aaseng: 27
AP Images: 11, 15, 21, 33, 36, 60, 65, 69
iStockphoto.com: 8 (bottom two), 55
Photos.com: 8 (top photo), 9
Science Photo Library: 39, 43, 48, 73

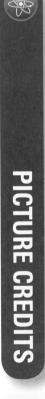

About the Author

Toney Allman holds degrees from Ohio State University and the University of Hawaii. She currently lives in Virginia, where she enjoys a rural lifestyle, as well as researching and writing about a variety of topics for students.

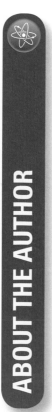